for Hayden and Talia

Elizabeth Borelli's
Beanalicious
Living

A Step-by-Step Guide to
Breaking Free from Processed Foods
and Embracing a Healthy,
Nutritious Lifestyle

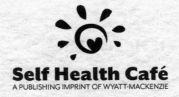

Self Health Café
A PUBLISHING IMPRINT OF WYATT-MACKENZIE

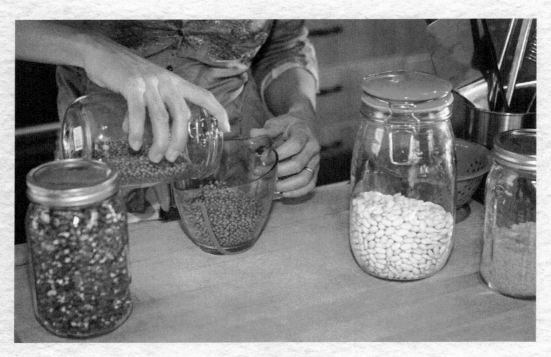

Beanalicious Living
A Step-by-Step Guide to Breaking Free from Processed Foods
and Embracing a Healthy, Nutritious Lifestyle

Elizabeth Borelli

Editing by Lisa Pliscou. Proofreading by Karen Kibler.

ISBN: 978-1-939288-19-6
Library of Congress Control Number: 2013939534

For bibliographic information visit www.ElizabethBorelli.com.

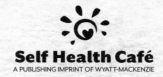

Self Health Café
A PUBLISHING IMPRINT OF WYATT-MACKENZIE

Contents

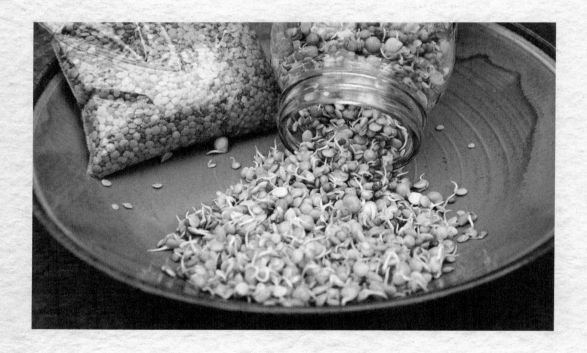

Introduction
Why Beans?

Way back in the day, our ancestors were hard-wired to hunt and to gather as many calories as they could just to survive. A lot of us now face the opposite problem: easy access to *too many* calories. And these days, processed food is much harder to *avoid* than it is to *amass*. As you can probably imagine, the statistics are disturbing. For starters, we consume 35% more packaged than fresh food, 95% of the grains we eat are refined, and close to 65% of Americans have at least one chronic diet-related health condition. Obesity, diabetes, heart disease— oh my!

So how do we tackle this dietary conundrum?

In a word: **beans**.

"Really?" you may be saying. "I'd like to be able to leave my house, at least on occasion!"

Never one to avoid the elephant in the room, I'll admit that beans do have a bit of a reputation. But it's one that is largely undeserved. This is one beneficial food group! And when you consider today's current options, beans' old-school reputation may be worth rethinking. In a society running on factory-produced foods—75% per meal on average— adding beans to your diet might start to make sense.

As a concerned mama and lover of all things healthy, I invite you to take a good, long look at your personal food portfolio: what you're eating, where it came from, and how it was made. Hint: none of this is obvious! While homemade oatmeal calls for three ingredients the McDonald's version uses 21 ingredients and contains more sugar than a Snickers bar. Clearly decoding food fact from fiction is no easy task. But it's so, so important.

This "what, where, and how" info is the basis for understanding how refined, processed foods affect not only our health, but our very well-being. Research conclusively connects our health, both physical and mental, directly to diet. As scientists are discovering, you really *are* what you eat. Food choices make a critical difference, and I believe it's time to think about some options. *Beanalicious Living* invites you to let go of the package for a moment and open your mind to healthy, whole foods, beginning with—but not limited to—delicious, nutritious beans.

While beans may be the red-headed stepchildren of the whole-foods diet, in reality they're amazing for so many reasons. Rich in protein, high in fiber, and low in saturated fat, these wonder foods are loaded with an unusually plentiful array of minerals and nutrients necessary for optimal health. Typically readily available, they're a cinch to prepare and when it comes to nutrients per calorie, beans are truly unbeatable.

A big part of *Beanalicious Living* is the story of how I unraveled my way from a processed-food stupor to discovering my inner kitchen ninja, with beans playing a starring role. But this adventure-turned-eating-guide is more than just beans. You'll find lots of user-friendly strategies for replacing our overly processed, fast-food diet with a healthy, delicious whole-foods version that's just as easy to follow and no more expensive. In other words, it's doable.

"But why change?" you may be asking. Packaged, processed food is easy, cheap, and pretty darn tasty, too (even if you only eat the "healthy" kind). So let me share with you some quick facts:

- **According to the U.S. Centers for Disease Control, more than one-third of U.S. adults (36%) and 17% of children (that's 12.5 million!) are obese.**

- **52% of kids' cereals contain more sugar per cup than three chocolate chip cookies.**

- **Obesity levels have climbed dramatically over the last 20 years, and are directly related to some of the most common health problems, including diabetes, cancer, and heart disease.**

beany bite

Beans are the only food to fit into two groups on the USDA Food Guide Pyramid: vegetable and protein.

Not only are beans versatile, studies confirm that including them in your diet, with their low caloric count and high fiber content, helps to lower cholesterol.

- Conclusive studies link the consumption of refined, processed food with obesity and related disease in both children and adults.

- U.S. Centers for Disease Control findings show that children and adults who eat fast food one or more times per week are at increased risk for obesity.

- Studies have found that people with a diet high in processed meats (such as hot dogs and bologna) had a 67% greater risk of developing pancreatic cancer than those who ate few or no meat products.

- Processed foods contribute to overeating and weight gain because you don't feel full as quickly as with high-fiber whole foods.

- The lack of fiber fails to slow sugar absorption into the blood-stream, so processed foods cause a spike, then a crash, in blood sugar levels—leaving you tired, hungry, and irritable—and, in the worst-case scenario, at risk for type 2 diabetes.

- According to the World Health Organization, processed foods are to blame for the increase in obesity levels and chronic disease around the world.

- To make up for the loss of nutrients during processing, synthetic vitamins and minerals are added to food to "enhance" nutritional content. The jury is still out on how often this really works.

- The word "Healthy" or "Natural" on a food package or label means absolutely nothing. According to the food-processing industry, all calories are healthy, and if an item contains water, you can check off that natural-ingredient requirement.

- Healthy, whole foods taste delicious, are easy to make, and are less expensive than refined foods when you prepare them yourself.

Just so you know, I haven't always been such a "bean queen"—in fact, far from it. Back in the day it was all about calories and taste, in that order, with fast and easy following close behind. My relationship with food was anything but healthy, but looking good from the outside was my number-one priority, and it didn't occur to me that feeling vibrant, energetic, and healthy could coexist with my version of fitness. Low-fat left me hungry, tired, and cranky, but I figured those were the choices: it was either stay thin or end up old and alone while people secretly made fun of my thighs.

Then, one day, my whole life changed—and my priorities along with it. *Hello,* motherhood! Suddenly it wasn't just about me anymore, and what a wake-up call. It became clear from day one that everything I did would have consequences that extended beyond me (no pressure!). I realized that a lot of the things I took for granted when I was younger and kid-less now needed further scrutiny when little ones were present. I needed to change my relationship with food, but first I had to do some fact-finding to find out how.

Looking at diet and lifestyle opened up a whole new world for me and for the two little girls whose health and well-being I'm responsible for. What started as concern and curiosity became a multi-year journey filled with fun and often frustration, but research and resolution prevailed. This book isn't about preaching, or scare tactics (although some of it *is* pretty scary)—this is about *empowerment*. Each of us is capable of controlling which substances, toxins, and pseudo-foods to let into our bodies; it's achievable with the smart-choice guidelines and user-friendly solutions in the Beanalicious lifestyle plan.

We'll begin with a look at some of the trickiest shenanigans happening right in our living rooms. I'm talking about TV (and other digital media). Advertising food to kids is big business, as in multibillion-dollar huge. And if your kids are watching, they're absolutely being influenced. As we'll see, none of us are overlooked when it comes to processed-food tactics and marketing schemes. It's not pretty, but I believe it's time to take a behind-the-scenes look at the industrial-food realities in order to make honest choices, whatever they are.

After an eye-opening journey through the dark side, we'll migrate

beany bite

Renowned health and wellness expert Dr. Andrew Weil recommends 1–2 servings of beans and legumes per day in his Anti-inflammatory Food Pyramid.

to greener pastures, or gardens as it were, to explore tips and tricks to help you make more nutritious food choices. The healthy food-preparation suggestions in *Beanalicious Living* are organized into clear-cut strategies for easy home cooking featuring beans, greens, and grains. Recipes are simple, options are endless: vegetarian, omnivore, flexitarian. You'll tailor ingredients to fit *you*, rather than the other way around.

The solution is clear: the food we eat is directly connected to our health, and fresh, whole foods are the way to go. Studies confirming the link between the American diet and lifestyle to our growing national health disaster are neither new nor surprising; we all know something's amiss and often, it's closer to home than we like to think.

The big question is, how do you know if you're making healthy dietary choices? Recommendations keep changing and it's hard to know what to believe. There's such a ginormous amount of health and nutrition news, tips, and information out there—who has the time to sort it all out? And even if we *had* the time to tackle that challenge, the bigger question for most of us is: can my crazy-busy lifestyle and a healthy diet even fit in the same sentence?

Whether these questions are on the tip of your tongue or anywhere near it, you're in the right place. Where step one is recognizing the problem, step two is talking solutions—solutions that are easily adaptable to your lifestyle, rewarding, and even fun. With this in mind, *Beanalicious Living* is not a "diet" in the Webster's sense. It's not calorie-restrictive, it's not food-specific, it's not short-term. Rather, it's a series of simple steps you can take on the road to healthier living without sacrificing money or time. It's a manual to help you take back your plate, one satisfying bite at a time, and have fun doing it.

I talked a minute ago about food and nutrition confusion. "Well then," you may be wondering, "where is all this confusion coming from? Who can you really believe?" These are great questions with big answers, all linking back to *what* you buy and *who* you buy it from. Our sneak peek into the industrial food business is sure to generate some "aha" moments; I think you'll like my suggestions for smarter, better alternatives.

Let's face it—when Walmart family founders control as much wealth as the entire lowest-earning third of our society, our culture has become one big infomercial. The pitch: consumerism; the promise: fulfillment; the price: disempowerment. And while this massive, complex problem has various possible fixes, none is so simple as taking back the plate. *Beanalicious Living* is a back-to-basics shopping, meal-planning, and preparation guide as the first step toward taking back our kitchens without losing our minds! And if you need a little help breaking free from the fat/salt/sugar cycle, I'm here to help.

This is awesome stuff, so let's get started. Your inner kitchen ninja is just a few beans away!

PART 1

Know Better,
Eat Better,
Feel Better

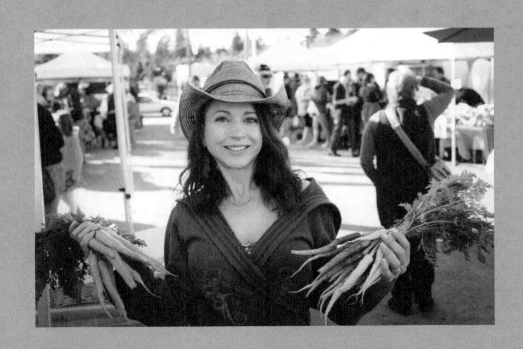

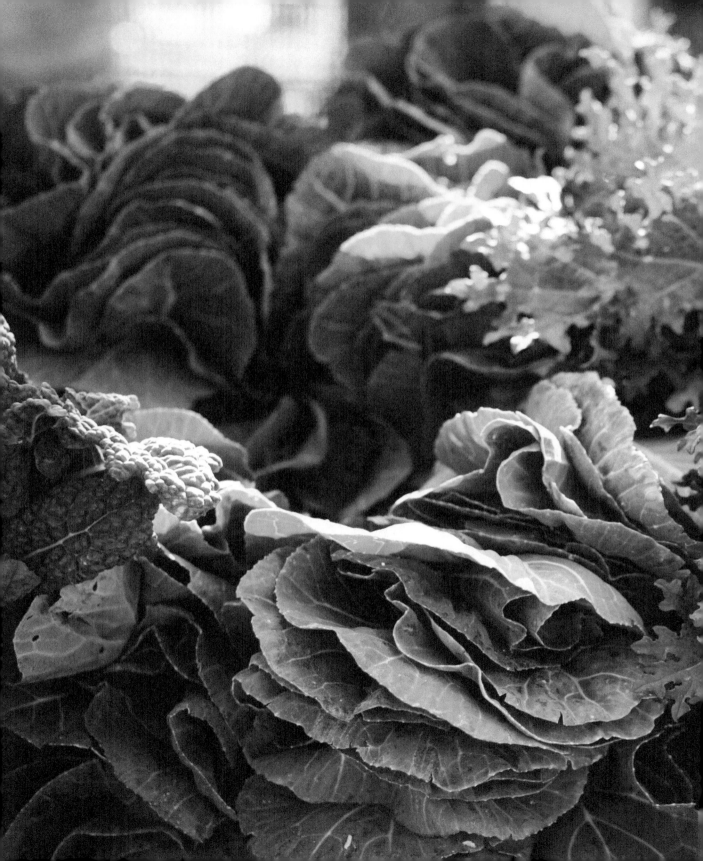

CHAPTER 1

Eating Outside the Box

It never fails. Every time I'm feeling sorry for myself because of some minor tragedy (or not enough yoga!), I'm always presented with a reality check. You know what I mean—you walk by someone in a wheelchair and suddenly you remember how lucky you are to have your health. It's true: good health tops the list of the basic prerequisites for happiness.

The problem is that right now Americans seem to have it all backwards. Health is on the decline as disease rates are on the rise, and there are no easy answers in sight. With studies conclusively confirming that food choices matter, our mentality isn't cutting the mustard when it comes to good nutrition. But the lack of a magic pill doesn't mean there's not a cure.

When it comes to eating right, a lot of us have it, well, all wrong. Sounds harsh, I know, but consider that 25% of us eat fast food every *day*! That's like spending every afternoon in a tanning booth and wondering why you're getting wrinkles. And even if you're ordering from the "healthy" menu, the question remains: whose definition of "healthy" are we hearing?

Most of us, regardless of how we decide to prioritize it, do care about achieving and/or maintaining good health. We're doing our best to opt for fat-free, avoid deep-fried, or pay a little more for the "natural" version. We're trying to save the artificially colored food for the occasional birthday or holiday. But . . . when the most visible information about which foods are called healthy is provided *and* promoted by the players with the deepest pockets, things really get confusing.

When most national food brands are owned by mega-corporations whose priority is keeping the bottom line healthy for their shareholders, as a consumer, you gotta wonder, who has our backs?

Most refined food is too high in all the bad stuff that's directly connected with our national rates of obesity and diet-related disease, but when it's being *advertised* as healthy, who wouldn't be confused?

At the same time, savvy food-industry marketers are out there promoting the next "healthier, tastier, skinnier" solution, even as diet-related healthcare costs keep steadily rising right alongside their fast-food profits. Talk about job security!

Despite the fact that 17,000 of these helpful new products are introduced each year, U.S. healthcare costs reached $2.6 trillion in 2010, 10 times the amount spent in 1980. What a conundrum! We've bought into a lifestyle that seems to demand fast, cheap, and easy, but these so-called solutions are making us sicker.

So to bring it all back home: what's a too-busy-to-research, more-into-eating-than-cooking, health-conscious mama to do?

When it comes to good health, you want to get it right, yet you barely manage a shower some days and on those rare occasions you find the time to tackle it, you're not even sure where to begin. Nutritional news is everywhere, ever-changing, and sometimes even contradictory. Is margarine good or bad these days? Depends on who you ask. Fresh studies crop up all the time, and new diet fads make the news regularly: high carb, low carb, no carb . . . .

It's become so bewildering that most of us have started to simply tune it all out, look for the labels "Healthy" and "Nutritious," and keep our fingers crossed. We just don't have time to decode the ingredients list, and who knows what half the stuff listed is anyway? "Monosodium glutamate? Must be a fancy word for salt—I'll take it!" Yes, it's easy to see how quick and easy (read "packaged and processed") often becomes the default.

But what if it didn't have to be this way? What if you had a plan that incorporated the most delicious, nutrient-intensive foods available that's *also* both time- and cost-effective? No, it's not a sale on

Slim-Fast. The big bad food industry has us all thinking their version of healthy is the only way to go. Wrong!

Enter the bean. The story of how whole, healthy foods have been marginalized and practically forgotten is a befitting narrative for our consumption-crazed lifestyle. Overreliance on overly processed has gotten us into this mess and it's no accident that we're bombarded with promotions, products, and pills promising to fix it. The sad fact is that it's profitable to treat the symptoms of this food-induced dilemma, and there's a whole slew of products to treat every one of them.

I used to wonder what was wrong with me—how could my one recommended serving of Special K with skim milk leave me famished just a short time later? Why, oh why, couldn't I be more like that peppy gal on the package? You may have guessed where I'm going here. Eventually I figured out that the superstar cereal eater doesn't exist in the real world, and it was time to begin searching for better nutrition—outside of the box.

Whether for health or environmental concerns, or even simply interest in one's appearance, it's increasingly clear to me that dietary changes are due, starting with limiting (and maybe eliminating) the number of quick and easy, tantalizingly promising, very processed foods that may have been getting you through your day. Here's the thing—no matter how convincing they sound, highly processed foods are never your best choices.

Yes, they'll tell you they're fortified, fat-free, and oh-so-good-for-you, but don't believe it for a minute. The words on the package aren't subject to a lot of regulation, leaving room for the rise of the phenomenon known in the marketing terminology of processed foods as the "halo effect." This sweet-sounding term is used to describe the positive impression terms like "Natural" or "Healthy" evoke when splashed across the package. Unfortunately those words can be used very deceptively and are therefore not necessarily true, but the halo effect influences shoppers into believing that products described that way must be good for us. And it's hard to believe some descriptions can deviate so far from reality. In the most obvious cases we're usually not surprised, but other times it can be downright disappointing. High-fructose corn syrup qualifies by the FDA as being "all-natural"—*really?*

Like most people, I'm not immune to the power of brand loyalty. My heart ached for days after learning about the high level of toxins that leach from the lining into the cans of one of my favorite all-natural, "homegrown" soups. It was my go-to brand; I had even blogged favorably about it! That was a real tipping point for me. I couldn't come to any other conclusion: processed foods simply can't be trusted, but the whole, fresh foods you prepare yourself won't let you down.

You may be thinking, "Cooking from scratch? Who does that anymore?" I admit that with a full schedule in one hand and takeout on speed dial in the other, it's hard to initially imagine life in an apron. But I'm here to tell you about the surprisingly minor amount of effort it takes to create a well-planned weekly menu. Start with a few simple basics; it will make a giant difference in your overall health and well-being.

Here's how I know. I've been focused on healthy eating for most of my adult life. I avoided fried foods and red meat, opted for low-fat whenever possible, chose wheat over white every time. And I tried to incorporate these choices into our family's cuisine. Yet despite these efforts my husband Neal still had high cholesterol and high blood pressure in his early forties; little Talia had asthma and my 10-year-old Hayden had difficulty focusing in school. Not exactly the portrait of health I was hoping for! Something was amiss. While at first I had no idea these problems were diet-related, I began to hear more and more about toxins found in many of the foods my family and I consumed on a daily basis, a fact which I found very disconcerting.

I'm neither a scientist nor a dietician. I began this journey as a concerned mom trying to avoid exposing my family to chemicals and food-processing by-products which are widely linked with disease. That's right—the same chemicals and processes that I used to think were regulated by the FDA or some other governmental organization . . . someone, *anyone.*

But I've since learned that many toxins are permitted for use in food products. Plus, manufacturers of those products are permitted

beany bite

One study which measured the effects of bean-eating on heart health found that people who ate legumes at least four times per week had a 22% lower risk of heart disease than people who ate them less than once per week.

to label them "Healthy," "Natural," "Good for you," or any description of choice except "Organic." Organic, as in associated with the USDA Organic Seal of Approval, is the only term required to have any true meaning or guidelines in food labeling today. No wonder we're confused.

I realized I needed to gain a broader understanding of the toxins lurking in the "health" food I was feeding my family. What began as a chemical-avoidance mission soon became an eye-opening expedition into smart nutritional choices, which—as it turns out—are quite different than the ones the government's "Food Guide Pyramid" publicly recommends. I decided to follow the proven research-based science of pioneers like Dr. Joel Fuhrman, Dr. Dean Ornish, and others, who advocate sensible, whole-foods eating instead of focusing solely on carbs, fats, or any other single nutrient that calls for a complete dietary overhaul that's unbalanced and difficult to maintain.

All this research was like opening a giant can of worms, or, in this case, beans. The more I learned about what goes on behind the scenes in our governmental food regulatory agencies, the more I realized we as consumers owe it to ourselves to maintain as much control over what we're putting into our bodies as possible. The more whole, unprocessed (and organic when possible) the better!

I know, I know—you don't have time to cook. Every minute is accounted for in our fast-paced society, and who wants to spend hours and hours slaving away in the kitchen? I agree! That's why I developed the Beanalicious planning tools and strategies. As a working mom of two, I didn't have time either. But the more I read, the more I learned, and the more I realized the critical role diet plays in health, energy level, and weight control, all of which are interrelated. Incorporating healthy whole foods into your life is a key part of that equation.

When I first started cooking from scratch, Neal was skeptical. "Seriously? You're going to stop buying canned food?" he said. "Why?" I couldn't blame him for asking. Why would anyone *not* buy the conveniently packaged foods we have so readily available? Well, the sodium, the hormone-disrupting chemicals in canned food liners, the waste, and the taste for starters.

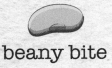

beany bite

One cup of cooked black beans contains 15 grams each of protein and dietary fiber, providing 30–50% of the recommended daily allowance—all for only 227 calories and less than 1 gram of fat.

And amazingly, as it turns out, cooking from scratch is not only cheaper, healthier, and more delicious, it's also inspired my family to a new level of culinary creativity. We've created so many fantastic dishes from the big batches of beans, grains, toppings, and sauces we whip up, it's become an endlessly rewarding adventure.

As a society, we've been marketed into believing that instant is essential to keeping our busy lives under control. We begin the day with boxed cereal and jarred juice. Lunch is fast, frozen, or packaged, and dinner is whatever you can pick up on the way home. The amount of fat, sugar, salt, and chemicals—regardless of health claims on the box—is far beyond anything that constitutes healthy, though you'd never guess it from the label. I sure didn't. The number of bottled smoothies I consumed during my pre–label deconstruction phase is too embarrassing to mention.

Yes, I bought into all that hype: pretty pictures of fruits and veggies that looked better than the ones in the produce section (no washing or peeling required), vitamins galore, and low-fat promises too good to pass up. I never looked on that tiny side panel which listed all the sugar, preservatives, and, oddly enough, very little real juice. Maybe I didn't want to know back then. Could a little sugar and a few additives really be all that bad? Rhetorical questions aside, the real issue is how misleading those claims are. When the truth is in fine print, it's pretty obvious what they don't want us to see.

The situation gets even stickier when foods promoted as "Pure and all-natural" contain mysterious additives with negative side effects. For example, consider carrageenan: it's an all-natural ingredient frequently found in both dairy and nondairy products to make them creamier. It's also known to cause inflammation and tummy troubles in some people, especially those with sensitive digestive systems like my daughter Talia.

Poor kid! It took me years to make the connection between our morning yogurt and the Tummy Tea that inevitably followed. Before I finally put two and two together, I thought it was a chronic problem I hoped she'd eventually outgrow. Had I known, through smarter shopping I might have been able to X out a line item on a future therapy bill!

beany bite

Beans, which unbeknownst to many are technically categorized as fruits, are one of the oldest cultivated crops in the world, dating all the way back to the Bronze Age.

We've become so addicted to this packaged-food diet and the remedies that often are then needed that, as Dr. Joel Fuhrman observes, "We can no longer tell the difference between health and health care." What I came to realize is that simply avoiding the *cause* of these ailments is the smartest solution.

Fortunately, the recipes I've compiled are so much better for you than the processed stuff that when you start to notice a difference in the way you feel, addictive patterns will start to shift. Positive habits can be addictive, too.

CHAPTER 2

Here's to Healthier Kids

Even as a longtime health vigilante, I still worry about my kids. American children are prime targets for Big Food, an industry that has the inside track to their attention through TV and every other form of media, played up to the hilt. These savvy folks are spending between $1.6 billion and $10 billion annually, depending on which source you reference.

Most of these ads are for junk foods—processed food loaded with calories, sugar, fat, and sodium. Show me a kid who doesn't harangue his poor mama for the latest cool character super snack food and I'll be worried. It's perfectly normal to really want something so awesome-sounding, especially when you're constantly being convinced that everyone else has it.

The Federal Trade Commission reported findings in 2006 that children ages 2–11 watch an average of 25,600 advertisements a year, of which 5,500 were for food and drinks. The most frequent ads were for restaurants and fast food, cereals (mostly sweetened), desserts, and other treats. So how does this shake out? Kids saw on average 1,400 ads for fast food and restaurants, 16 ads for vegetables and legumes (the Jolly Green kind), and not a single ad for fresh fruit.

The American Psychological Association reports that most kids under the age of eight don't differentiate TV from reality, which makes them the ideal audience. Since advertising works by repetition, with fewer than 100 TV ads per year that kids see for healthy whole foods, it's clear who's got the mindshare here. (P.S. It's not the tofu!)

These pricey tactics are clearly working and the results are nothing

beany bite

A traditional form of Indian medicine, Ayurveda is translated to mean "the science of life." This 5,000-year-old system emphasizes the importance of good nutrition, including legumes, which are often present in every meal of the day.

short of disturbing. American kids are bulking up. As I've mentioned, numerous studies conclusively tie diet to obesity-related disease. So when the U.S. Centers for Disease Control and Prevention reports that the percentage of obese children ages 6–11 in the United States has almost tripled since 1980, we have bigger issues than just oversized children.

A number of obesity-related diseases such as high cholesterol and type 2 diabetes are also on the rise. Type 2 diabetes, formerly known as "adult onset diabetes" (a term which, for obvious reasons, no longer works), is now at epidemic levels among children. But surprisingly, it doesn't behave the same way it does in adults. Type 2 diabetes progresses faster in kids than in adults and is harder to treat. Add that to the fact that obese children are significantly more likely to become obese adults, and go on to consider the serious health and social issues that come with that—and I ask you, what's a health-conscious mama to do?

One thing's for sure: we're not going to change the system, at least not anytime soon. I'm no Nancy Negative, but the fact that the food and beverage sector is a $1.5 trillion industry renders it highly unlikely they'll stop pimping their processed party foods voluntarily.

While studies conclude that both advertising and availability of processed junk foods directly correlate to obesity in children, this information is promptly dismissed by Big Food. A representative from the food industry lobbying group Center for Consumer Freedom clearly explains their position: "[Our strategy] is to shoot the messenger. We've got to attack [activists'] credibility as spokespersons." Unfortunately, this was not a recap of a *Sopranos* episode—it's lobbying as usual, and worse still, it seems to be working.

Here's an illustration: Americans are now spending over 140 billion dollars a year on fast food, a figure that increases annually. The average five-year-old consumes 64.6 pounds of added sugar each year, 60% more than his or her body weight. And while the Big Food industry assures us there are no bad foods, a McDonald's cheeseburger Happy Meal with fries and soda contains two times the amount of fat and calories recommended *for the entire day*. So for now, it's up to us to get the facts and make smart choices, even under imminent threats of a public tantrum over that box of Lucky Charms.

But let's focus on the bright side: we're lucky to have information on and access to a bold new way of eating—or, to put it another way, a return to the simpler foods we knew and loved before we were lured into this quagmire. Those of us with children have the opportunity to develop young allies, and with a little education, kids really get it! My 10-year-old daughter Hayden has been overheard matter-of-factly explaining to friends that commercials are created for one reason only: to convince people to buy things they really don't need, and sometimes aren't even good for them. Who could argue with that?

I talk to both of my kids about industry advertising and nutrition statistics in ways that make sense to them. I keep it short and to the point and try not to come across like the teacher in the *Peanuts* specials! We'll talk about how even though that smiley box of macaroni and cheese looks so inviting, the "Yellow 5 and 6" it contains are artificial food dyes linked to attention deficit hyperactivity disorder in children. My kids know what goes into McDonald's hamburgers and prize or no prize, they have no interest in going there.

I'm not suggesting you scare your child away from all treats or turn them into paranoid food-conspiracy theorists, but it's good to let them know there are two sides to the story: yours and the commercial food industry's. I once asked the influential activist and author John Robbins what inspired his commitment to campaigning for the ethical treatment of animals. He shared his recollection of a poster that hung on the wall of each of his family's Baskin-Robbins stores, showing happy cows in a green sunny field. His firsthand knowledge of the super-sized discrepancy between truth and advertising created an "aha" moment that inspired his epic work, and he's among the small (but growing) number of advocates putting health before profit.

I like the idea of sharing with kids the underrepresented, noncommercial nutrition information that's not obvious unless you seek it out. The American Academy of Pediatrics has an informative website where you can order magazines created for kids designed to engage them in ways they relate to. Organizations such as Spoons Across America

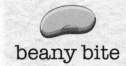

beany bite

A recent study shows that bean-eaters weigh on average 7 pounds less and had slimmer waistlines than non–bean-eaters—even though the bean-eaters consumed nearly 200 calories more per day.

offer food and nutrition education information for kids as well.

There are also great whole-foods cookbooks for kids. And while neither of my girls are budding Rachael Rays, almost every day Hayden whips up a mean and healthy smoothie loaded with fresh fruit and a bit of stevia for extra sweetness. Snacks like homemade granola or apples topped with fresh peanut butter are a cinch to prepare and refreshingly free of hidden sugars, unhealthy additives, and saturated fats. I've found that if you can get kids to grow it, make it, or even pick it out, chances are they'll make friends with foods they would otherwise avoid.

When I need to, I can always find an alternative that works. Most kids love snacks like fresh fruit, banana chips, nutty trail mix, and edamame. It may not be their first choice if they're used to a shiny package, but when most yogurts, granola bars, juices, and cereals come with ubiquitous high-fructose corn syrup (HFCS), which has been directly linked to obesity, I urge you to make the switch. However, I also must warn you that this can be a process requiring patience, experimentation, and mistakes. At first you're likely to hit some resistance, which could include the classic "But everyone else gets it!" Yes, the majority of the people *do* get this kind of stuff, and that's the problem. But we can start to fix the problem—in our own homes.

For starters, consider replacing the need for speed with the urge to read—the label, that is. HFCS is the big red flag on ingredient labels and you'll find it on the majority of processed snacks aimed at kids. I recommend you avoid it. Despite glorious pictures of whole fresh fruits and exciting nutrition claims, if the label shows that it contains unhealthy additives like HFCS, saturated fat, or food coloring, then it probably isn't your best choice.

It's hard to overemphasize the importance of carefully reading the labels on packaged foods, even if you need to bring along your magnifying glass to be able to see them. "The Nutritious Choice" so confidently proclaimed on that package of Lunchables may cause you to overlook the 67 different ingredients, including many impossible to pronounce, listed in fine print on the side. We'll talk more about label reading in Chapter 12, "Nutrition Label Shakedown," but for now just suffice it to say, don't ever believe anything you read on the front of the package!

And once you know which ingredients to look out for—as in *include* or *avoid*—it becomes easy to incorporate healthier alternatives without a personal chef or a degree in culinary arts. Lots of times it's an easy switch: a different brand or version. Other situations can be more challenging, but those are often the most urgent.

For example: my friend Kimberly reluctantly agreed to let her son bring his teenage friend along for a weekend away. Her reluctance was due to this young man's reputation as a wound-up, rather obnoxious fellow. As it turned out, this boy had a regular drinking habit: sports beverages. The kind that have lots of bright tattoo art on the cans. One look at the label and my friend put the kibosh on that. An interesting day later, a whole new kid emerged. The link between diet and behavior, especially in children, is well documented.

The dietary habits we establish as children often stay with us for the rest of our lives, so whole-foods, low-sugar, whole-grain, and little unsaturated fat are the way to go. Let's continue on our fact-finding journey in the next chapter, "The Frenemy on Your Plate," and when we get to Part 2, "The Beanalicious Solution," I've got some delicious, kid-friendly recipes to share that I guarantee you and your family will love.

beany bite

Beans for your brain: electrolytes such as the potassium found in black beans are minerals that help your body maintain a healthy system, including optimal brain function.

CHAPTER 3

The Frenemy on Your Plate

It's hard to ignore the inconvenient truth: the American diet is due for a major makeover. Our waistlines keep expanding as the rate of diet-related disease continues to grow to epidemic proportions. Surplus money and leisure time seem to be the only things shrinking in this unfortunate scenario.

So is it the fat, the carbs, or the calories that cause all the problems? The diet industry has built a multibillion-dollar business by focusing on each of these culprits interchangeably, depending on their latest so-called cure. Yet, if that's the case, why aren't any of these packaged solutions or diet-restrictive meal plans ultimately working?

Nearly 65% of dieters return to their pre-diet weight within three years, according to Gary Foster at the University of Pennsylvania's Weight and Eating Disorders Program. Moreover, only 5% of people who lose weight on a calorie-restrictive diet (such as a liquid diet or a no-carb diet) keep the weight off long-term.

Are Americans just a bunch of gluttons who lack self-control entirely? Or are we simply overextended—not sure where to begin and overwhelmed by it all? Sadly, it's the status quo we can blame: fast, easy, and disguised as healthy is both the default and the problem. Fortunately for all of us there is hope, because regardless of what Jenny Craig says, it's not only *how much* we're eating, it's *what* we're eating: mainly processed, refined, and factory-farmed foods.

You may be thinking, "If this explanation is really legit, why aren't more people aware of it?" And that, dear reader, requires a little history of what we're up against. Big hair wasn't the only product of the eighties. It's been three decades since the USDA first stepped up to take a stab at offering the nation some nutritional advice. Our government was hoping to address the rising rates of diet-related disease, which add to our economy woes in the form of higher healthcare costs. With much ado and plenty of outside influence, the Food Pyramid was born. Unfortunately for us, the USDA walks a fine line where these recommendations are concerned.

Consider the fact that the USDA is the acronym of the U.S. Department of *Agriculture*, not the U.S. Dietary Association—which is the role they've assumed when they published their perky pyramid. So I ask you this: when the department in charge of aiding and abetting the agricultural industry offers food suggestions, how conservative do you think they're going to be? That fine line is starting to look more like a rubber band—stretching to fit Big Ag demands while still managing the task of rendering advice of some sort.

Tricky business, but the USDA was able to eventually concoct what in its wisdom it saw as a satisfactory solution. Since the Big Food industry does not take kindly to its products being called out for bad behavior, it was able to convince the USDA to adopt its crafty mantra: all food contains calories; we need a certain number of calories to live; therefore, there are no bad foods.

So instead of advising avoiding or substituting—two dirty words in Big Ag-ville—the creators of the pyramid just decided to, well, *include*. In other words, the Pyramid plan okays your regular drive-through habit as long as you meet the rest of your daily food-group recommendations, which is by all definitions a whole lot of food.

Today, the Food Pyramid has morphed, with a few minor updates, into MyPlate, but the "Eat more" advice remains the same. It's not hard to imagine how the supersize was born. If you followed all of the Pyramid/MyPlate serving sizes and food group recommendations, you'd be well on your way to bigger before you know it.

None of this has gone unnoticed in the academic community, where doctors and researchers also want to get to the widening bottom of this problem. Both the Food Pyramid and MyPlate endured tremendous criticism from some very potent sources. For example, faculty members at the Harvard School of Public Health created a new Healthy Eating Pyramid, which offers easy-to-apply rules of thumb as shown in an accompanying Healthy Eating Plate. These guidelines are strictly based upon 20 years of academic science and nutrition studies. More importantly, they use words like "less" and "avoid" when they need to.

I don't know about you, but when offered the option of a Harvard-researched solution or a Big Ag–influenced one, the choice seems as clear as the beans on my plate. Interestingly, both the USDA and the Harvard dietary guidelines stress the importance of a plant-based diet, but only the Harvard guidelines expressly advise avoiding processed meats and high-fructose corn syrup, and limiting things like white rice and potatoes.

More on that later, but the point here is that both the very conservative USDA guidelines and the science-based, progressive Harvard School of Public Health recommendations advise reliance upon a plant-based diet, which means reduced use of processed and takeout foods and more fresh, home-prepared whole foods.

This is doable. Really! I know all the excuses—I've made them myself. "No time, too expensive, it's too hard! Maybe slaving away in the kitchen was fine in the fifties, when June stayed in the kitchen while Ward was at work and the Beav kept himself entertained outdoors all day. That's not my life; I'm too busy to cook." And so on.

It took me years to learn what I needed to change, and more years still to figure out how to change it. There's no one-word answer, but in the spot-on words of best-selling author and wellness advocate Kathy Freston, we can start by *leaning into it.*

Some steps are easy, like identifying the worst of the processed offenders and replacing them with healthier, no-cooking-required alternatives. For example, when my savvy niece Emma learned that her all-time favorite crackers contained trans fats, she promptly switched them for carrot sticks. Still crunchy, still orange, and a whole lot better for her.

Not everyone can make this kind of dramatic switch. But when you know what to look for, you can stave off a snack food craving with

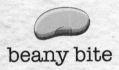

beany bite

Acclaimed nutrition expert and best-selling author Dr. Joel Fuhrman describes beans as the best choice for healthy carbohydrates.

a healthy alternative, like organic cheese popcorn—assuming it passes your nutrition-label inspection, of course—to replace those low-fat cheese puffs, and it's no more expensive or time-consuming. Eventually you may find time to make your own snacks or figure out some fruits and veggies that will suffice, but you can start by leaning in, one step at a time.

When it comes to healthy diet, it's all in the planning. Few of us have the willpower to resist the frenemies in our cabinets, never mind on our plates. My recommendation? Don't let them in! A recent *New York Times* study found that five years after the California school junk-food ban was introduced, which simply limited accessibility at lunchtime, students are consuming fewer fats, sugar, and empty calories on a daily basis than when that stuff was readily available: 158 fewer calories on average, which may not sound like much initially, but in the long term, it adds up to a pretty significant reduction.

It can be as simple as out of sight, out of mind. Researchers say that most of us could avoid significant long-term weight gain by cutting out just 100 to 200 extra calories a day, which as any dieter knows is much easier when no one is dangling a bag of chips in your face at lunchtime!

Little tricks like planning ahead, creating a list, and sticking to it are basic first steps in the process. So hang in there—in the chapters that follow I'll walk you through just how to do it.

beany bite

Beans are good for your hair. It's true! Aside from their high levels of protein, which promote hair growth, beans offer ample iron, zinc, and biotin—all nutrients supporting healthy locks.

CHAPTER 4

Diet, Delusion, and Billion-Dollar Business

Ever wonder why you can't flip through your favorite "women's" magazine and avoid the latest diet trend news? In spite of diligent calorie-counting and love of all things low-fat, adult obesity rates increased in 31 states in 2012. At 34% nationally, the stats are already too high. And yet you can't turn a corner without bumping into the latest wonder fat blaster. How is this happening?

Just think about it: every time you walk by a newsstand, turn on the TV, or go online, you see it. It's like a weight-loss minefield! If you didn't feel self-conscious before, you probably do now. And everyone wants to sell you the magic antidote. Delicious, satisfying, and *this* time, they swear to everything holy, it's for real. Sometimes they even have a sexy celebrity to back it up. It all sounds so convincing—who wouldn't want to try it?

Sure, some of these fad diets and over-the-counter cures do result in weight loss initially, and who doesn't love the fun and positive attention that comes with it? But if you're anything like 90–95% of the population, those excess pounds will return, and with them the feelings of failure; not only did you fail, you failed publicly. I've ridden that wave many times, and believe me when I say it's no fun.

But the thing I didn't realize back in the eighties when I stuck religiously to the high-protein diet—a *big* trend that decade—is that healthy weight doesn't come from shame, denial, and endless calorie counting (thank goodness). I'm relieved, and excited, to be able to share truly

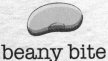

beany bite

Beans make you feel good! They contain a variety of minerals as well as the B vitamins that are associated with decreasing anxiety and depression.

enjoyable options with you. After years in the trenches followed by years of research, I say: It's time to be nice to ourselves!

Our national weight increase keeps lots of companies in business, but personally I'd rather see economic gains focused on healthier solutions than those that come in a package. Americans spend more than 37 billion dollars on dieting and related products every year. To put it into perspective, we spend 40% more money trying to lose weight than we do on national security—and for all of our sakes, let's hope our national security programs are more effective! But if any of these so-called solutions actually worked, the scale would be tipping in the other direction.

Instead it's just the opposite. We're in the midst of a diet/health crisis that is more than just a result of happenstance, weak willpower, or planetary misalignment. Certain entities are working diligently to influence our dietary choices and melodramatic as that sounds, it's the simple truth. When customers stay hooked on processed, packaged foods, they keep both manufacturers and the diet industry in booming business.

As nutrition expert and author Marion Nestle remarks, "At the supermarket you exercise freedom of choice and personal responsibility every time you put an item in your shopping cart, but massive efforts have gone into making it more convenient and desirable for you to choose some products rather than others." These massive efforts—in the form of designer packaging, sexy celebrities, and enticing promises—lure us in. And who can blame us for wanting what Heidi Klum calls healthy when we've craving a little snack . . . and that package of Fat-free Fruit Flirtations, with her smiling face on the front, is right there within reach?

It is no exaggeration to state that billions of dollars each year go into convincing us that the tens of thousands of processed-food products contain special key nutrients or miracle ingredients that will transform us into slim and healthy hotties. Unfortunately, most of us don't read past the front-panel proclamations to the tiny fine print which tells the real story, so we buy it!

Is it really legal for companies to make claims that aren't true? The

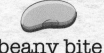

beany bite

Health magazine named black beans as the leading superfood for weight loss. *A cup of black beans contains an impressive 15 grams of protein, so it keeps you satiated longer without the unhealthy saturated fat found in animal-protein sources.*

Nutrition and Education Act of 1990 legalized the use of claims on food packaging that promote the relationship between a nutrient or food and a disease or health-related condition. So when you see things like "Helps reduce risk of osteoporosis" on a product to which a drop of calcium has been added, the finished product doesn't even have to be tested to see whether that's true. So in general, if there's any way it could *possibly* be true, no matter how remote that possibility, it's okay to say it.

Big Food is indeed a huge industry with tremendous influence: from the farm to the factory to the halls of Congress, they've got it covered.

However, I want to make it clear that I'm not suggesting *all* processed food is bad. Much of it does have its place in the pantry—I'm pretty sure most of us aren't interesting in grinding our own corn—but the fact is, most processed foods are refined to the point of eliminating the natural nutrients, then combined with dubious ingredients and chemicals that have the potential for creating serious health problems.

Let me introduce you to the Beanalicious **"Foods to Avoid"** short-list: the processed foods you might want to keep off your shopping list. They:

- contain ingredients you don't recognize and usually can't pronounce
- contain GMOs, BPA, HFCS (we'll talk about these creepy acronyms in Chapter 8)
- contain high levels of sugar, sodium, and saturated fat
- contain food additives, dyes, and preservatives
- always come in a package

So now that we've outlined what's wise to steer clear of, the next question is: what are the *healthy* foods?

There are lots of different opinions on this subject, and I've spent an enormous amount of time researching them—which led me all the way through a Cornell certificate program in plant-based nutrition based on the work of eminent scholar Dr. T. Colin Campbell.

Nutrition is a huge and multifaceted topic; the jury is still out on

beany bite

Got antioxidants? Small red beans are the #1 food source, but red kidney beans contain high levels as well. Antioxidants protect cells from free-radical damage, which has been linked to cancer and other chronic diseases.

many of the issues, and legitimate-sounding studies seem available to back every point of view. Fortunately, there *are* islands of certainty within these stormy waters. A visit to Food Fact Island #1 reveals that processed foods—especially those containing high-fructose corn syrup and/or high levels of sugar, sodium, chemicals, and/or preservatives—are not only unhealthy, but are contributing to weight gain.

Studies show that on average, a full one-third of our daily calories comes from nutritionally deficient processed foods such as processed snacks and fruit juices. That means 30% of our food is just empty calories—empty except for the fat, sugar, and chemicals, that is. Did you know that 22 million Americans eat at McDonald's *every day?* But the equation doesn't end here: our overall daily food intake is also on the rise. So despite all the low-cal, fat-free versions of just about everything we now have available, we're eating 25% more calories today than we did in 1970. Any way you slice it, more empty calories, plus more overall calories, adds up to overweight.

Sail on over to Food Fact Island #2 and discover that, according to a growing number of experts, Americans are eating too much meat, and it's contributing to our obesity and diet-related health problems. In spite of the disturbing evidence, people in the US continue to consume on average ½ pound of meat per day.

So why aren't we getting the message? Maybe because the message has become so confusing! The meat industry works very effectively to promote meat as being synonymous with protein, and it's the first thing most people worry about when those veggies beckon: "But how will I get enough protein?"

According to our friendly factory farmers—you'll learn more about them in Chapter 10—if we're not extremely diligent in our meat-eating, before we know it we'll be withered, anemic, and too weak to reach for the cheesesteak we *should* have eaten, had we only listened to them.

The irony is that not only is protein from meat not superior to vegetable protein, meat is *also* synonymous with the troubling practice of factory farming—at least 99% of it is. Funny how in all the "facts" Big Food loves to feed us, they forget to mention that part.

beany bite

One cup of cooked beans meets 25% of the recommended daily allowance for amino acids, along with more calcium and iron and fewer calories (without cholesterol!) than 3 ounces of cooked meat.

The reality is that Americans have little to worry about in the protein department; we're exceeding U.S. government standard recommendations there, too. Fear not, dear reader! You'll never become protein-deficient with a whole-foods diet rich in beans, grains, and good leafy greens. They've got you covered . . . just without all the saturated fat.

I've mentioned one of the biggest signs of trouble in our society: the growing rate of obesity and diet-related diseases in kids. Talk about getting off to a bad start! According to the Centers for Disease Control and Prevention, approximately 17% (or 12.5 million) of children and adolescents aged 2–19 years old are obese. And this number is growing! As I've also mentioned, kids who are obese are at higher risk for serious health problems, such as type 2 diabetes, heart disease, and asthma rates—which are also on the rise. Scary stuff!

Last year alone, the biggest food companies spent tens of millions of dollars lobbying on Capitol Hill, with more than $37 million used in the fight *against* junk-food marketing guidelines for kids. Recent statistics show that nearly 70% of food advertising promotes the least healthy foods out there: convenience foods, sugary treats, soda, and alcohol, while a measly 2.2% is allocated to fruits, vegetables, grains, and beans. Do these companies really think they're making our jobs as parents easier? Clearly they're not run by people who take their kids grocery shopping.

The fact is, plenty of us are eating more of everything *except* the right things. Super-sized portions, the kind you see offered at every fast-food counter, are only available for low-quality, empty-calorie foods. It's a lucrative opportunity for manufacturers to charge an extra 50 cents for another cup of soda that costs them 5 cents. Of course they're pushing it.

The bottom line? In our society, we're constantly enticed to fill up on empty calories and too much meat, yet we're still not getting the nutrients we really need. The good news is that since they're empty anyway, it's pretty easy to switch those refined grains, simple carbs, and factory-farmed meats for flavorful alternatives like the beans, grains, and greens so abundant in the Beanalicious lifestyle.

beany bite

Beans are a great source of magnesium, a mineral shown to relax the nervous system and stabilize blood circulation, and is great for keeping both mental and physical fatigue at bay.

Here's the skinny: fresh, toxin-free foods are not only delicious, they'll make you healthy, too. "Up to 75% of our health destiny is determined by our daily diet and lifestyle choices," says Dr. Andrew Weil, wellness expert, best-selling author, and founder of the Arizona Center for Integrative Medicine at the University of Arizona. So if our destiny isn't primarily predetermined by family history, we have lots of opportunity for improvement— starting with our diet!

CHAPTER 5

Tricks, Tactics, and Intentional Confusion

So . . . just why *is* nutrition information so confusing?

With all the constantly changing, often directly contradictory information out there, it's becoming more difficult to—putting it in food terms—weed out the wheat from the chaff. Are dietary requirements for the human species really constantly changing? Is science truly making new nutritional finds all the time? In a word, no.

General, scientifically based nutritional guidelines and recommendations for preventing diet-related disease have hardly changed in the past 60 years. *Eat a greater variety of foods including more fruits, vegetables, whole grains, and legumes. Restrict intake of calories, fats, sugar, and salt— in other words, less of the nutrient-deficient stuff.*

This nutritional advice still rings true today. Of course, we've made critical advances in science and medicine that are helping people to live longer—an amazing achievement—but while our lifespans are increasing, our health is decreasing earlier than ever before. In essence, we're allocating more and more of our precious time on this planet to living with illness, thanks in large part to our modern food system.

You may be wondering, "Are healthier options *really* that hard to come by? And if they're not, why aren't they more widely promoted and publicized?" This conundrum begs the question: who could possibly stand to benefit from a nation of junk-food eaters?

As it turns out, the list of industries that cash in on disease and illness is long: prescription-drug companies, diet-pill pushers, lipo

beany bite

Beans were so revered among the ancient Romans that the four most distinguished families were named after them: Fabius (fava bean), Lentulus (lentil), Piso (pea), and Cicero (chickpea).

doctors, even specialized lingerie companies like Spanx (the one I personally can't dismiss out of hand!) . . . on and on it goes. But again, if these so-called solutions really worked, why is the problem getting worse and not better?

I'll tell you why. Because there is one option that, while optimally effective and doable by just about everyone, is sadly unsung. That solution is simple, whole-foods, plant-based eating. Fresh, whole foods will never gain the media-darling status of processed foods for one reason: no process, no profit. Direct from the local farm cuts out the industry altogether.

Farmer Joe down the road isn't out there pitching his home-grown peas as the next hot superfood; we *know* fresh organic peas are good for us no matter who grew them. There's little profit to be made in prevention; but as long as we're overweight and unhealthy, industry cashes in, which remains their primary objective.

Let's take a closer look at the sprawling U.S. food industry, comprised of companies that produce, process, sell, and serve food, beverages, and dietary supplements. It's a trillion- dollar industry accounting for about 15% of our annual GNP. It's *huge.* And as we all know, mammoth corporations need to keep those profits growing to keep their stockholders happy. This might be all well and good if they had a growing market to keep up with production, but that is simply not the case.

The behemoth U.S. food industry is so incredibly efficient, it currently produces nearly twice as much food in the form of calories per capita as we need. It's a staggering demonstration of the economic syndrome of marketplace over-competition, driving producers to become ever more creative to get you to buy their goods instead of someone else's.

Enter the "Eat more" messaging: *Got milk? How about protein? Vitamin-enriched, nutrient-fortified, anyone?* And guess where these marketing efforts are focused. That's right—they're pushing the products that bring in the biggest profit. Whether they're good or bad for us is, from an industry perspective, irrelevant.

The more processing stages a product is pushed through, the

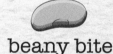

beany bite

Beans are a good source of heart-healthy fiber. Black beans in particular stand out because of their high antioxidant levels, which also help to strengthen the immune system.

more revenue opportunities are available, and usually, the ingredients that go into the product are the cheapest ones the company can source. It can cost more for a manufacturer to *package* a snack food than it costs to make the product itself! And often the lowest-quality foods are the ones most ardently touted; since they cost the least to make, they fetch the biggest profit.

As Marion Nestle comments: "Food companies will make and market any product that sells, regardless of its nutritional value or its effect on health." I find this pretty scary, don't you? Most of us assume that food products are carefully regulated by the government, so that the public isn't duped into buying unhealthy food based on misleading health claims—a tactic which should rightfully fall into the false advertising category. However, this is far from the case.

But where is this tricky messaging coming from? If it's not accurate, how can it be so flagrantly promoted?

To get to the root of those questions, we need a better understanding of who makes the rules and how they're implemented.

The common element among all of Big Food's behind-the-scenes food production practices is the compromise of public health and nutrition in order to maximize profits. At first glance, this might seem like a page from *Elementary Business 101.* Food manufacturers are in the business of making new food products and getting us to buy them so they can make money, of course!

It's the *how* of it that's unsettling. Consider, for example, my friend Farmer Joe down the road. Suppose Joe decides his peas should be sweeter and better able to resist pests, so he takes his seeds into a lab and creates a new SuperPea, which he markets as extra-sweet and healthy. It looks to us like a regular pea, only greener and more perfect. The problem is that no one knows what those fancy lab tricks will do to us in the long run. And although Farmer Joe doesn't know the long-term effects either, that's not what he's telling us, because he's not required to reveal that kind of processing information to consumers.

When it comes to processed food, a cookie is never just a cookie. As a society we've become so disconnected from our food production, we don't even know what we're eating anymore. But we need to. The rise in popularity of the work of whole-foods proponents like author, journalist, and activist Michael Pollan reveals an exciting, growing trend toward an interest in incorporating more healthy, locally grown whole foods into our diet. However, we've outsourced so many of our food-preparation practices to Uncle Ben, Mrs. Butterworth, and Betty Crocker, we're not sure how to take it back.

The good news is, it's easy to relearn those old-style techniques, and you'll be amazed at how much better you'll feel as you develop your new relationship with food and nutrition. And good, wholesome food is something to love. For every tempting Dorito, there's a sweet, juicy Concord grape!

While there are lots of factors contributing to our nation's dietary woes, in my opinion one of the worst is having junk food thrust in our faces while friendly voices tell us how healthy it is—and there's no one really representing the alternatives. So I was delighted to read a new report released by the National Institute of Medicine which recommends limiting junk-food marketing to children and boosting the availability of healthy foods as a priority measure to improve public health.

The fact is, when kids are consistently being convinced that processed food is linked to fun and even social acceptance, and given easy access, they'll choose it over healthy food, which they just know as, well, healthy (read *borrring!*). Salty, fatty, and sugary foods are addictive, and who knows what the added chemicals do? Kids make the perfect target market, since they tend to think in the immediate, believe what they're told, and as for willpower, that's a tough one for any of us.

I know that a lot of this is hard to take in. I've been there. As a mom I've had long-term love affairs with many a boxed cereal, only to find out the pitch was based on half-truths at best. It's a sad day when you realize you can no longer feel good about feeding your kids cereal for breakfast, and it's not even the fluorescent or sugary kind. Personally, I was horrified to recently learn that the cereal I lived on while pregnant with Talia—because it was fortified with folic acid—actually exposed me to an additive potentially linked with cancer. While I was later relieved to learn the folic acid claim was disproven, you get my point. Food claims should not be taken at face value;

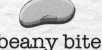

beany bite

Beans are good for the earth! According to scientists, legumes are capable of fixing atmospheric nitrogen. In layman's terms, this means that legumes replenish nitrogen in the soil, enriching it for future use.

beany bite

Beans contain the amino acid tryptophan, which helps to regulate appetite, aid in sleep, and even reduce symptoms of depression.

there's almost always another side.

This would indeed be bad news if there was no light at the end of the tunnel. Fortunately, it's easy to replace those processed foods with real, whole foods your kids will actually enjoy. And here's looking at the issue from another angle: the goals you have for your family are in all likelihood very different from the goals of the companies selling you processed foods. In fact, you might say they're pretty much at odds with each other.

Aside from you, the ones who benefit most from your healthier eating choices are small farmers and local producers, neither of which controls advertising budgets that put them in the same league as Big Ag and Big Food. The challenge is to seek out smart nutritional information for yourself . . . while the food industry spends $37 billion a year telling you not to worry, they've got your back.

The reality is that the behind-the-scenes work of the Big Food conglomerates influences most of what we believe about good nutrition today. Get this: the largest food companies such as Kraft and Nabisco were founded or purchased by big *tobacco* companies. No wonder their tactics sound so familiar! With so much money and influence on the table, the regulations become subject to lots of varying interests which, in turn, seems to result in a lot of creative-rule bending, especially when it comes to product labeling.

As industry analyst and author Michele Simon notes in her eye-opening book *Appetite for Profit*, industry follows trends, good or bad, and diligently works them to their advantage. That box of Lucky Charms enthusiastically touts the trusted "whole grains" promise despite the fact the cereal contains less than 1 gram of fiber per serving and is lacking in essential nutrients of any kind.

And don't those impressive promises on the package sound too good to be true? Well, they *are* too good to be true. The maddening part is, they always seem to know precisely what to say. Just look at any one of the alluring magazines lining the checkout counter and you know who they're playing to: we all want more energy, sexier abs, and a youthful glow, so that's what our food-product advertisers promise to deliver.

Meanwhile, a full 95% of the grains that comprise the American diet are the unhealthy refined kind—which have been implicated in raising the blood fats, called triglycerides, that put you on the fast track for a heart attack or stroke. Despite all the glowing claims, good health rarely comes from a package. Bummer, huh? If the insta-meal that truly rivaled fresh and whole was out there, I'd be all over it.

I'm all for choosing the time-saving solution, but we have to draw the line when it jeopardizes our health and wellness. Yes, there are those occasional compromises we need to make to save some sanity. When faced with a snarlingly hungry seven-year-old and no fruit salad in sight, I'll go for the granola bar every time, heck with the sugar content. But I make that the exception, not the norm. It's impossible for me to forget that the chemicals and additives in processed food affect us in ways we might not even realize. Whole foods beat processed for nutritional value every time. My family and I are living proof of that.

For years I suffered from blood sugar spikes and dives; they were caused by a diet of too many refined carbs. I hadn't realized that my energy bars, smoothies, and processed snacks were the cause of the problem. I would crash to the point of falling asleep in the middle of the day—and it never occurred to me to look at my diet.

Discovering the prolonged energy effects of beans and whole grains has changed my life. I'm always ready to exercise. Closing in on 50, I'm stronger than I've ever been in my life, much more alert, and just plain happier. And I've sworn off caffeine for good because I no longer need it. I'll never go back to eating foods that make me feel bad, and my only regret is arriving so late to the party. Which begs the question: why don't more people know about this?

Industry advertisers dish out up to 50 times the amount the USDA spends on promoting the MyPlate nutritional eating guidelines and encouraging people to eat whole foods. As I mentioned in Chapter 1, healthy-sounding descriptions like "All-natural," "Fresh," and "Nutritious" have no real meaning, nor are there any USDA or other defining guidelines they need to follow. "Low-fat," for example, enthusiastically touted as a healthy alternative to the standard fare, turns out to be another cagey term. (More on this in Chapter 14.)

The USDA allows manufacturers to list "qualified health claims" or similar statements on a food label, accompanied by an explanation such as the limited amount of scientific support for their claim. For example, the front of the label might say, "Pomegranate juice reduces your risk of heart disease," followed by an asterisk. Elsewhere on the label, the disclaimer might say, "This claim about pomegranate juice has not been scientifically proven, and is based on limited evidence from rats." Terrific. And how many of us can read type that small anyway?

This is tricky business. When the big ol' companies whose campaign contributions let them weigh in on matters that could affect them negatively, rules tend to get bent. These guys are pros at keeping the laws as industry-friendly as possible. After all, a little dioxin here and there won't kill you . . . will it? In this day and age, the answer is "Not until you can prove it."

So we're being told which foods to eat by the people who profit from them, and who are allowed to reference studies that aren't scientifically valid which they use as proof of their health claims. Have you heard the one about yogurt helping with weight loss? Dairy producers sold a whole lotta high-fructose corn syrup–sweetened yogurt before they were reined in with a major lawsuit for that one.

Every packaged food out there comes with a promise, usually one telling you how good it is. The official industry line on the subject? "Any food that supplies calories *or* nutrients should be recognized as useful in a nutritious diet." In other words, there are no bad foods— just ignore those silly carcinogens.

Or you can try the alternative: fresh, healthy, home-cooked goodness. Once you take the time to learn the ropes, home-cooked will seem like the new normal. And pretty soon, you won't have it any other way.

CHAPTER 6

Adventures in Healthy Eating

So there I was, a determined mama on a chemical-avoidance mission—with two young children, a hectic schedule, and a long daily commute added into the mix. I would frequently return home in the evening to a cold, messy house with my kids in tow. I'd walk into the kitchen to find that day's breakfast dishes looming, homework and piano practice imminent, and no plan for dinner in place. I wanted to buck and run, thinking the kids would eventually be motivated enough by basic survival needs to pitch in and help out. Instead they just whined.

I began talking with other moms I knew and it turns out I was not alone. In fact, the more friends, acquaintances, neighbors, and family members I spoke with, the more I realized I'd stumbled upon a theme: overwhelmed is the new normal.

You've heard me say it before: a lot of us are in need of a diet makeover. This is not news. Each year, we the people rely more and more on processed and fast foods, even as we're warned over and over of the troublesome side effects from all the excess sodium, chemicals, and saturated fats they contain. As a report summarizing a recent Harvard debate on the subject proclaims, "Judged by its impact on health, the American food supply is a disaster."

Yikes! Are we *trying* to avoid being healthy? Or are we just too busy and bewildered to think about it? The good news is, while with diet and nutrition there are no easy answers, it doesn't have to be rocket science either.

I'm here to tell you that the road to wellness can be wonderfully

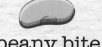

beany bite

Want to avoid type 2 diabetes? Introduce more magnesium-rich foods into your diet, such as beans, greens, and whole grains.

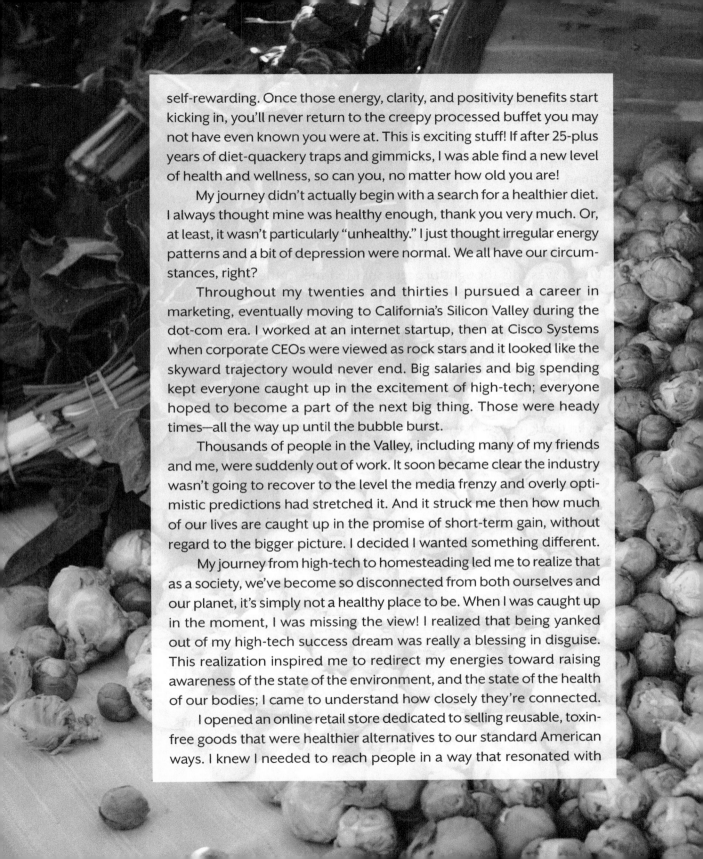

self-rewarding. Once those energy, clarity, and positivity benefits start kicking in, you'll never return to the creepy processed buffet you may not have even known you were at. This is exciting stuff! If after 25-plus years of diet-quackery traps and gimmicks, I was able find a new level of health and wellness, so can you, no matter how old you are!

My journey didn't actually begin with a search for a healthier diet. I always thought mine was healthy enough, thank you very much. Or, at least, it wasn't particularly "unhealthy." I just thought irregular energy patterns and a bit of depression were normal. We all have our circumstances, right?

Throughout my twenties and thirties I pursued a career in marketing, eventually moving to California's Silicon Valley during the dot-com era. I worked at an internet startup, then at Cisco Systems when corporate CEOs were viewed as rock stars and it looked like the skyward trajectory would never end. Big salaries and big spending kept everyone caught up in the excitement of high-tech; everyone hoped to become a part of the next big thing. Those were heady times—all the way up until the bubble burst.

Thousands of people in the Valley, including many of my friends and me, were suddenly out of work. It soon became clear the industry wasn't going to recover to the level the media frenzy and overly optimistic predictions had stretched it. And it struck me then how much of our lives are caught up in the promise of short-term gain, without regard to the bigger picture. I decided I wanted something different.

My journey from high-tech to homesteading led me to realize that as a society, we've become so disconnected from both ourselves and our planet, it's simply not a healthy place to be. When I was caught up in the moment, I was missing the view! I realized that being yanked out of my high-tech success dream was really a blessing in disguise. This realization inspired me to redirect my energies toward raising awareness of the state of the environment, and the state of the health of our bodies; I came to understand how closely they're connected.

I opened an online retail store dedicated to selling reusable, toxin-free goods that were healthier alternatives to our standard American ways. I knew I needed to reach people in a way that resonated with them, and hoped to better help them connect to the message through carefully selected products. Yet eventually that too seemed, well, contrived.

The "green" label became more and more of a widening marketing trend until it was clear to me that many people were, in fact, missing the point. Sustainable living isn't about using the right products or even eating the right foods; it's about *bringing it home*. It's about jumping off the commercial treadmill that has us ramped up to earn more so we can consume more. It's about taking back control of our lives.

It was this thought process that led me to the work of John Robbins. I mentioned him in Chapter 2—if you're not familiar with Robbins' story, I highly recommend you check it out. Formerly the sole heir to the Baskin-Robbins ice cream fortune, he walked away in search of a more fulfilling lifestyle than he felt that path could offer. What Robbins learned during his time with the largest family-owned ice-cream enterprise on the planet is that big business isn't always up-front with customers. It's become the norm to "Let the buyer beware"— even though most of the time the buyer doesn't even know what to look out for. Is high-fructose corn syrup *really* just like sugar? How many of us have the answers?

This decade-spanning search-and-discovery mission led to me delve deeper—not just into healthy eating, but one that also includes lifestyle changes that work long-term. Studies show that lots of the diet plans out there work in the short term, but very few have staying power because most are based on deprivation. And as most of us know, it's what you feel you're missing that you tend to focus on. As healthy eating expert and author Geneen Roth remarks, "For every diet there's an equal and opposite binge."

Realizing that diets and junk food just don't work, my next step was finding the healthier alternatives I needed to replace the processed ones. I tried supplements and superfoods, plus all things raw, juiced, and fermented. I've spent hours in classes and many more in the kitchen, enjoying the results . . . and also testing my sanity to the limits. I like to cook, but still, all that time in the kitchen was making me a little, well, nuts.

beany bite

Multiple studies have linked bean consumption to a reduced risk of heart disease, type 2 diabetes, high blood pressure, and breast and colon cancers.

Where processed doesn't work, neither will complicated, at least for most people. Real, lasting lifestyle changes take place when there are good (or better) alternatives that produce a favorable outcome. I've learned a lot about this topic and how to migrate toward a healthier, happier way of eating. Let's dive a little deeper.

Because change is best embodied as a process, and because I want you to succeed, I'm not going to recommend that you drastically alter your lifestyle in any way that hurts. Instead I invite you to try cooking whole, natural foods like beans and grains from scratch. Think about introducing a new dish into your diet once a week to begin. And every week, one step at a time, you'll ease your way gently back to the basics. Before you know it, you'll find that by cooking just two pots of beans per week, you'll have the main ingredients for six easy, healthy, delicious meals each week.

There are tons of books currently on the market advocating certain specific methods of eating. There's the caveman diet, which, as you might expect, includes lots of meat-based protein; the Beauty Detox diet, where animal products, all refined foods, and even legumes are off limits; and countless diets for all points in between. Many of them have merit, having effectively shown significant widespread results in claims of lowered weight loss and improved health. Indeed, when researchers compared three popular diets for weight-loss efficacy, results among them were surprisingly similar.

It turns out the common success factor among them was adding more fiber-rich legumes and veggies as well as reducing sugar from the dieter's daily intake. While these diets vary in their choice of protein options and which foods to avoid, they all have one thing in common. Every medically validated food regime advocates or insists upon eliminating processed foods.

That's right. Replacing processed foods with healthier alternatives seems to be the common denominator among most diet and weight-loss programs, especially those not requiring use of special foods or supplements (as do Weight Watchers and Slim-Fast).

My education and research have inspired my recommendation to reduce meat and dairy products in your diet as much as possible

beany bite

Did you know that legumes are a good source of calcium? And since the calcium in legumes doesn't bind with its plant protein—unlike the calcium in dairy products—it's also easier for your body to absorb.

and replace them with whole-food, plant-based alternatives including, but not limited to—you guessed it—beans. A review of eating plans that actually work long-term shows that concentrating on the whole-food, plant-based approach is the surest way to reach your health and weight goals. And that's without swearing off meat or dairy, counting calories, or adding a crazy exercise regime.

For most of us it's doable, and with a few simple guidelines and the *Beanalicious Living* strategy to guide you, it can be an adventure with all kinds of exciting returns.

But no matter which health advice you choose to adopt, you'll probably need to do more home cooking to implement it. Now, I realize that for some, this is not necessarily good news, at least in the beginning. I had to start from scratch, just like you may have to. Meal planning and preparation can sound intimidating if it's new to you. The key—as in so many lifestyle improvements—is to make a plan that *works for you*. Ease in gradually, and before you know it, you'll forget you'd ever done it any other way.

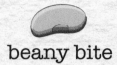

beany bite

Jazzy! The legendary Louis Armstrong was also a legume-lover extraordinaire. Lest anyone forget it, he signed all his letters "Red beans and ricely yours."

CHAPTER 7

Industrial Food: Even Worse Than It Sounds

Nutritional issues aside, from a consumer's perspective, our current food-distribution model is a disaster waiting to happen. Remember the banking crisis, during which a few large corporations controlling most of the home-mortgage market gamed the system so that they all profited and ultimately, we all paid the price? Well, industrial food is looking scarily similar. Over the past 30 years, there's been a massive consolidation of our food-processing and distribution system as a smaller number of huge corporations gain control over more and more of our food chain.

I'm no conspiracy theorist, and no, the sky isn't falling, but given some of the issues this country has faced when we let monopolies run amok, the following facts are worth considering:

- Of the 40,000 food items in a typical U.S. grocery store, more than half are now brought to us by just 10 corporations.
- More than 90% of soybean seeds and 80% of corn seeds used in the U.S. are sold by *just one company:* Monsanto. Three companies—Monsanto, DuPont, and Syngenta—own 47% of the world's seeds. And they own 65% of the global corn market.
- Four companies are responsible for up to 90% of the global trade in grain.
- Nearly every major food commodity—including wheat, corn, and soy—is controlled by just four corporations.
- Today, three companies process more than 70% of all U.S. beef: Tyson, Cargill, and JBS.

And what do corporations do when they're in control of a market? Yep—these guys are on the job, cutting corners and bending the rules to squeeze out more drops of profit than an orange has juice. It's easy to add a few "nutrients" to a feeble mix of ingredients, then spend millions telling us how healthy it is. Of course, the message is never "Stop eating processed food" as the solution for the diet-induced illnesses vexing our nation; instead it's "Try this *new* processed food" as the cure. This pernicious loop leads to an endless array of new products, more profits, and the same old problems never addressed.

Let me clarify that this isn't an anti-business, down-with-profits rant. I'm all for success in business and that rightfully involves making money. But . . . .

As far back as 1992, food companies have practically revolted every time the Department of Health and Human Services released new dietary guidelines; they've loudly condemned the advice gleaned from a consensus of government and private-sector scientists and nutritionists as "too restrictive." This advice included limiting intake of certain foods, such as saturated fat, sugar, cholesterol, dairy, and meat. Pressure from Big Food resulted in watered-down guidelines that, even though the recurring dietary themes of *Eat more plant foods and less animal and processed foods* have been the same for the past 70 years, are about as straightforward as, um, a multi-committee, government agency report.

So if you remember nothing else about this highly abridged history of the USDA Food Guide Pyramid, keep this in mind: the advice that served as the backbone for the original Pyramid could have been boiled down to these simple words: *Eat more plant foods, fewer animal and processed foods.* Now, following industry uproar, voluminous discussion, and the passage of several decades, we have something akin to this: *Don't worry about limiting anything, just be sure you're covering all of the food groups.* In other words, eat more.

And it's working. As a nation we're averaging 10–12 pounds more weight since the Pyramid was first put into place. That's enough to increase the cost of traveling by $5 billion a year for additional jet fuel to fly heavier passengers, and $4 billion annually to cover additional gasoline costs to carry heavier passengers by car. A study released in 2012 by the Campaign to End Obesity estimates that the cost to treat obesity adds an additional $190 billion a year to U.S. medical costs. Do we *really* believe finding the magic "nutritionally fortified," low-fat, low-carb packaged food is going to fix things?

Unfortunately, a lot of us do believe it. As processed-food consumption has risen, over the past 30 years we've seen a 300% increase in type 2 diabetes in children. Coupled with alarming rises in cardiovascular diseases in younger kids, and predictions of shorter life expectancies for American children for the first time in our country's history, we've got a fight on our hands.

Our best weapon? Our forks!

We need fresh, whole foods in place of processed junk—even the dubious stuff labeled "Healthy." I stopped buying packaged cereals for my kids years ago, even before there was so much information available about the dangers of processed foods. I had learned from a nutritionist about the cereal extrusion process and how there's almost no recognizable part of the original ingredients left in the final product. Not good. So I stopped (pardon the pun) cold turkey and switched to homemade oatmeal, fruit smoothies, and whole-grain cereals and breads. *Voilà!* Out with the sugar, in with the fiber, and on to begin a healthy new day.

Of course my kids protested at first. But they realized they actually *liked* the new foods I was introducing. They got used to this new style of eating and now they've practically forgotten there's any other way to eat. I talk to them very directly about how businesses need to make as much profit as possible to be successful, and if you can't really tell what's in a food product by looking at it, the people who make it have lots of opportunity to tell you what you want to hear. Of course it says on the box it's healthy in bold yellow letters! But as nutritionist and food-label expert Jeff Novick advises, *never* believe the claims you read on the front of the box.

In my family, it helps that our journey to healthier eating has been a gradual one. Now that nutritious is our new normal, we don't have to freak out when occasionally it isn't. I know full well when everyone else is guzzling Mountain Dew at the sleepover, my kid will imbibe and I don't make a huge deal out of it—but I make sure it's the exception, not the norm. Think of it this way: you wouldn't let your child eat food off the floor, even if there's only a one in a hundred chance they'll catch something from it. These days, when one in two people has either diabetes or pre-diabetes, it's actually riskier to eat out of the package— especially when you take the long view of your child's health and future.

Since 2005, studies have been linking diabetes with Alzheimer's disease; more recently, this association has been reexamined, even making headlines among the likes of mainstreamers like Dr. Oz. New research offers increasing evidence that takes this connection from coincidental to causal, with poor diet being named a main culprit. In fact, people who have diabetes also have twice the risk of developing this scary degenerative condition.

While we now know that diabetes doesn't cause dementia, they both stem from the same source: unhealthy diet. Ominous as that sounds, the upside is that scary diseases like Alzheimer's may not develop so randomly after all, and we can choose alternatives that lower our risk factors considerably. Kind of makes whole foods taste all that much sweeter if you ask me.

Where Big Food and Big Ag are concerned, we know they're up to no good—but as long as we keep buying their products, they have no reason to change. Again, this isn't a vendetta against corporations per se; they're doing what they need to do to keep their profit margins growing. In fact, it's their legal responsibility to their shareholders. But . . . it's the grand scale of the misleading information campaigns, lulling us into a false sense of trust, that make this mama mad.

Big Ag has the big bucks, while the little guy, the family farmer, not so much. And the ensuing loss of thousands of family farms, the pollution of air and water, and growing health epidemics that result from Big Food business practices deserves to be recognized. The playing field is so uneven, it makes the board game Monopoly seem fair. More and more frequently, the choices that determine which foods

beany bite

Beans are the most budget-friendly source of protein available. Cooked beans contain 12–14 grams per cup; cooked lentils weigh in at a whopping 18 grams per cup.

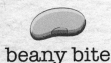

beany bite

Variety is the spice of life: currently, the world's gene banks hold about 40,000 different bean varieties. However, only a fraction are mass-produced for regular consumption.

appear on our supermarket shelves are made by corporations pretending to be a mama's best friend, while sapping her mojo without her even knowing.

This is troubling in more ways than one, dear reader. We all deserve access to the healthy, fresh, and chem-free foods our small farmers provide us with bountiful variety. Thank goodness we have more options than just good old iceberg. But offering variety in fresh, time-sensitive food reduces profit for Big Food. So industrial food companies leave us with fewer, compromised, and more expensive choices. When profit is the driver, the cheapest to grow or manufacture wins out over quality every time.

Compare the variety of your local farmers' market to that of even the biggest grocery store, and there's no contest. I don't need 75 varieties of snack chips but I do want more than two varieties of tomato to choose from, and the only way to ensure that is to support a wider variety of suppliers. Every time we buy our food from a small farm either directly or through one of their local distributors, we vote with our dollars for a strong, independent food supply. I love my food too much to have it commoditized. I hope you feel that way, too.

CHAPTER 8

Why Organic?
HFCS, BPA, and Other Scary Acronyms Best Avoided

I've been talking about all kinds of things we're better off not eating. While I think it's smart to avoid overindulging in any rich food on a regular basis, it's sinister synthetics we really need to watch out for. From the lab to our plates, these chemicals and by-products are hidden in most processed foods, and although most of them are widely recognized as potential health threats, you'd never know it from the labels.

Just pick up a box of breakfast cereal, and notice the lovely, natural-looking, and perfectly toasted corn flakes featured on the front. Sprinkled among the flakes you'll see some delicious fresh fruit (not included) along with some cheery words about fortified vitamins and minerals and how good this cereal is for you. A healthy breakfast choice, right? That's what I always thought.

Okay, I used to reassure myself, *maybe it's not the health-nut choice, but at least it's not bad for me.* And I'm no longer embarrassed to admit that even when I did look at the ingredients, I had no idea what those 20-letter words meant. But it's breakfast cereal, for God's sake, and what else are you gonna have time to eat before starting your busy day, right?

Wrong.

We can use the power of the fork to say, "No more!" Because now we know that when we see that this breakfast food contains high-fructose corn syrup (HFCS) as a primary ingredient, we'll know it's a red flag and drop this cereal, or any other packaged food containing that toxic ingredient. Because now we know it's linked to the other, behind-the-scenes red-flag ingredient: genetically modified organisms (GMOs), which are present in 95% of the non-organic corn on the market today. I was shocked to discover that, and maybe you are, too. But information is power, and we're here to get our game on, so let's keep going.

Once we know we need to read beyond the front of the box, the next thing we need to know is how to understand the secret code. Actually, it's not really secret—it's just not obvious. Even the most health-conscious consumers experience the mass confusion that is natural-foods labeling. What do these terms like "All-natural" and "Organic" really mean, and who can we trust to tell us?

While the water at first seems muddy, a few simple tips will render it crystal-clear. There are only a handful of descriptors you can count on not to have been bastardized to all shades of gray by food-industry lobbyists. One of most widely used of these is the word "Organic."

Here's the Wikipedia version: "Organic foods are foods that are produced using methods that do not involve modern synthetic inputs such as synthetic pesticides and chemical fertilizers. Organic foods also do not contain genetically modified organisms, and are not processed using irradiation, industrial solvents, or chemical food additives." This is what the USDA food-labeling guarantees. So while use of the word "Organic" doesn't always translate to super-nutritious—many processed organic foods still contain plenty of sugar and fat—you're at least avoiding those modern synthetic ingredients that are truly the worst of the lot.

Packaged foods proudly proclaiming the "Natural" label are often made from products grown using synthetic pesticides and chemical fertilizers as mentioned above. Plus, as if that's not bad enough, these tricky "natural" foods usually contain the hidden ingredient I alluded to earlier: GMOs, which are not allowed in organic foods, but are not required to be identified on the label, so unless it's organic, you can't know for sure.

Fortunately—and this is where the "information is power" part really comes into play—GMOs can be detected using another easy method. Since GMOs have managed to find their way into 95% of the corn supply, they're pretty much always present in high-fructose corn syrup. HFCS is in the majority of processed foods because it's the cheapest and most readily available sweetener, thanks to all the government corn subsidies.

So of course the lightly sweetened corn flakes contain GMOs, as do most yogurts, salad dressings, crackers, snack foods, and fruit juices. Mind-blowing, isn't it? And we thought we were making *healthy* choices. So let's take a closer look at some of these additives, and why I recommend that you avoid them.

Genetically Modified Organisms

Strolling through the aisles of most grocery stores, it's hard to believe that an estimated 80% of the packaged foods will contain GMOs. But you'd never know that by looking; the government hasn't required labeling because it doesn't want to "suggest or imply that GM/GE foods are in any way different from other foods."

The odd part is, the studies claim truth on both sides. Even though industry-sponsored studies *all* claim their GMO-infused foods are no different from non-GMO foods, independent studies often show they are—and right now no one knows for sure. GMOs haven't been around long enough for us to determine that. And since our government has opted to go with letting the buyer beware instead of requiring conclusive test results, why not take a little time to understand what it is you need to be aware of?

First off, what *is* a GMO? Think of it as a whole new breed of organism made by manipulating genes from one species—like bacteria, plants, or animals—into another to introduce a new trait, such as longer shelf life in produce, greater pest resistance in plants, or to manipulate an increase in the production of meat and dairy items.

So why would this concern us? New improvements make things better, don't they? In this case, my belief is probably not. While there may be compelling opinions supporting each side of the GMO debate, genetically modified organisms are part of a relatively new field of experimentation, which means all the facts are not yet available.

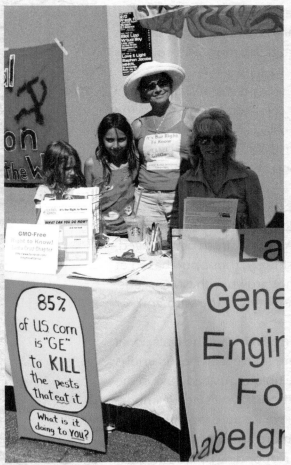

The real effects of GMOs on humans and the environment may not be known for decades. In 1992, the Food and Drug Administration officially proclaimed a lack of any evidence showing that GM foods were substantially different from conventionally grown foods and therefore were safe to eat. This reassuring claim was subsequently challenged by a lawsuit which publicized internal memos showing that their position was staged by political appointees under direction from the White House to promote GMOs.

Dr. Jeffrey Smith, a leading author and expert on the subject, identifies numerous studies linking GMOs to a number of negative health effects, including increase in allergenic reactions and damage to virtually every organ studied in lab animals. The American Academy of Environmental Medicine plainly states, "Genetically modified foods have not been properly tested and pose a serious health risk."

The FDA's own scientists have warned that GMOs can create unpredictable, hard-to-detect side effects, including allergies, toxins, new diseases, and nutritional problems. Despite these scientists' insistence that long-term safety studies were needed before GMO products were introduced into the public food system, this advice was ignored. Add that to the fact that all of the European Union and dozens of other countries require labeling of any product containing genetically modified ingredients—isn't it curious why in the U.S. we have no such regulation?

As crazy as it sounds and despite the fact that 90% of people polled have let our government know that *we want to know,* these foods are not required to be labeled. Yep, even though health and environmental risk factors have been clearly identified, big business is keeping pressure on the FDA not to require labeling, and so far it's worked.

But then again, who knows? GMO seeds, plants, and products—although they require more pesticides and aren't living up to the promise of ending world hunger—may actually turn out to be perfectly healthy to eat, or at least not unhealthy. Wouldn't that be great! But . . . we still want to know. In my opinion, it's the *not knowing* that raises the biggest red flag.

In case you're ready to go hide under the covers at this point and not come out, please don't. Remember, knowledge is power, and for you and me this situation is correctable. Any food, fresh or packaged, that's labeled "Organic"—as well as, most likely, those purchased at your local farm or farmers' market—are not grown with GMO seeds. (Whew!) If it's not labeled "Organic," and if it *is* made with corn or soybeans, it probably contains GMOs.

Does this mean you're risking your life by nibbling the occasional GMO corn chip? I'm guessing if that were so we'd all be in various states of decay by now. But I do put these ubiquitous bad guys in the "best avoided" category. Unfortunately, these days it's nearly impossible to avoid them altogether, but I believe it's sure worth it to try. The good news is, as shoppers become more aware of these issues, some food manufacturers are voluntarily responding by labeling their GMO-free foods accordingly. This helps when you're looking for all-natural popcorn that really *is* as good as it looks.

High-fructose Corn Syrup

Waistlines have been widening ever since high-fructose corn syrup, or HFCS, started secretly sweetening our lives around 30 years ago. With a slightly higher fructose level than sugar, HFCS does much of its damage because it's hidden in so many places you don't expect to find it.

So what's the problem? It's just a little added sugar, right? Not according to recent studies. Researchers from the University of

Southern California and the University of Oxford have discovered a link between rates of diabetes and HFCS consumption. They studied the rate of HFCS consumed in the food supply in 42 different countries, the U.S. topping the list with an average of 55 pounds per person per year. Countries that consume more HFCS have higher rates of type 2 diabetes than low consumers, such as France, Japan, and Italy, where average consumption per person is one pound or less.

A Princeton University study compared high-fructose corn syrup to fructose (regular white sugar). Researchers found that rats fed HFCS-sweetened water over a six-month period gained 48% more weight than rats given the sugar-sweetened version, even though their diets and caloric intake were otherwise the same.

What's worse, the HFCS group developed symptoms of metabolic syndrome, often a precursor to diabetes, which makes sense given the new findings. You've probably heard some of the confusing claims that HFCS is just fine: it's all-natural and the recurring health concerns are all hype, but like much of the nutrition news out there, it's important to consider the source.

When Big Food finances the studies, is it a surprise when the results go their way? HFCS is in many packaged products, and it's directly linked to the growing rates of obesity and diabetes in this country. But given that HFCS is so much cheaper to produce than regular sugar, regardless of the problems this unhealthy additive is creating, it's not going anywhere soon.

This makes even more sense when you look at how modern industrial agriculture developed in the U.S. Way back in the day, during the time of the Great Depression, farms were mostly small and independently owned. With so many people unable to afford to buy food, the farms responsible for feeding them were struggling to stay afloat. Our government came to the rescue in the form of cash subsidies, as in free money paid out to farmers for growing certain crops, which ensured the farmers' commitment regardless of whether the crops were profitable in the consumer market. These subsidies have stayed on the books since then, but the landscape under which they were written sure has changed.

Now instead of keeping our farms in business, our taxpayer dollars are hard at work tilting the growing fields in favor of certain single-species plantings, or monocrops. Corn and soybeans, those GMO darlings, are the crops the most heavily subsidized in this muddled equation. These cash contributions have made HFCS cheap to manufacture, and with all that extra sweetness it brings to packaged foods, it's an industrial food producer's dream come true. So it's added to lots and lots of items, and as a result the foods that are most processed are also the least expensive.

If I had a magic good-health wand, I would wave it and switch those subsidies from monocrops (which lead straight to the production of HFCS) to fresh fruits and vegetables, and shower those farmers with funds to make sure they stayed profitable, so they too could lower prices and level the playing field. Wouldn't that be great? We could afford to eat more of the fresh produce so essential to good health—instead of the junk food that's causing so many problems—and the farmers would make a fair profit. Sadly, there is no such wand, and this notion remains a fairy tale. Consumer prices on processed foods are increasing at *half* the rate of fresh fruits and vegetables, which economies of scale and government subsidies keep low. No wonder so many hungry mamas reach for the high-voltage energy bar and not the fresh fruit bowl.

As I've discussed, our personal health is closely linked to the food we eat. The food we eat is directly tied to an industrial agriculture system that rewards giant corporations with billions of dollars annually, enabling them to produce things like genetically modified corn to use as sweeteners, fillers, and by-products in processed foods. The hard part for consumers is that HFCS has found its way into so many things we generally assume to be healthy, even items like whole-wheat bread. And as long as the label says "Whole Wheat, All Natural," what's wrong with a bit of sweetness in your wheat bread?

Nothing—if only it came without the side effects. But one of the big commercial benefits of corn syrup is that it allows food to remain on the shelves longer without spoiling. And because it comes from corn, it can be labeled "Natural" despite the fact that it's heavily processed during the manufacturing process. So already your "Whole Wheat, All Natural" bread is losing points in the healthy-food department.

Another serious problem with HCFS is that it inhibits the production of leptin, a hormone produced by our fat cells that tells us we're full and to stop eating. Studies have shown significant weight gain among subjects who substituted HFCS for sugar in otherwise identical diets, as these subjects experienced an *increase in appetite*. You heard me right. The low-fat yogurts and salad dressings that are supposed to keep us slim and trim contain ingredients that make us hungrier.

So, once again, we've got to ask ourselves the hard questions. Are food manufacturers *really* trying to help us get healthy, or are they just saying whatever we want to hear to get us to buy their products? If the term "pusher" comes to mind as an answer, you're not far off.

Recent research suggests that foods sweetened with either sugar or HFCS can be as addictive as nicotine or narcotics. Sounds extreme, doesn't it? But it's sure something to think about. Sugar, along with alcohol, nicotine, and caffeine, are the four highest-volume items sold in grocery stores.

Remember the big interest in the French mystique—all those best-selling cookbooks and self-help books? Did it make you wonder how those French women stay so thin with all that wine, cheese, and pastry? Perhaps it's because they know what they're eating—and it isn't being chemically enhanced, genetically modified, and laden with corn syrup. As I mentioned a little while ago, the average American eats 55 pounds of HFCS per year; a typical French person consumes only *one pound* a year.

Lest it sound like I'm extolling the virtues of processed cane sugar in my vendetta against the evil HFCS, I'm not. I'm suggesting eliminating foods containing HFCS wherever possible *and* reducing the amount of sugar in your diet—thus avoiding exposure to all of the scary side effects. Remember how I mentioned in Chapter 2 that the diets we adopt as children tend to follow us into adulthood? It's never too early to change direction and usher out those processed foods . . . *tout de suite.*

Bisphenol A

Here's one more stealthy processed food by-product you need to know about: Bisphenol A (BPA). This sneaky compound is a hormone-disrupting chemical which can mimic estrogen, and has been shown to produce negative effects in animal studies. You may remember back in 2008, BPA became big news when the dangerous levels found in baby bottles prompted a mass recall.

That was good news for babies and all was quiet on the BPA front, right up until 2010 when the FDA released a report that raised further concerns about BPA exposure to fetuses, babies, and kids. Soon after that, Canada was first to declare BPA a toxic substance. France and China soon followed with major steps in regulating or outright banning this controversial chemical commonly found in plastics such as food containers, canned-food linings, and even in cash register receipts. That's all fine, but what about here in the U.S.?

Frederick vom Saal, a scientist and expert in the field of developmental biology, explains the situation like this: "The Japanese industry voluntarily removed BPA from can linings 10 years ago and thus, were able to reduce exposure to BPA by 50 percent. Last year, Congress asked companies in the United States to take similar actions; however, companies have made no move toward compliance." In spite of this, the FDA still has no official plan to ban BPA from consumer goods.

According to vom Saal, babies exposed to BPA while in the womb are at an increased risk for obesity. This isn't a new theory, since BPA has been linked to obesity risks in numerous other studies. Some researchers estimate that exposure to BPA generates double the insulin production that people need to break down food. Higher insulin levels are linked to issues like obesity and type 2 diabetes. But how much exposure to BPA are we actually getting from these brief encounters? A recent study showed that eating a can of Progresso soup caused levels of bodily BPA to jump 1,000%, and that varying amounts are present in almost all canned foods.

This problem is one of the biggest reasons I advocate cooking beans from scratch. I discovered the amazing health benefits of beans long before I became focused on avoiding many of the more serious toxins present in food, so for years I made chili, hummus, and salads with canned beans. They were convenient and tasty, and seemed much easier than preparing beans from scratch. But now that I'm a soak-and-stovetop convert, I'll never go back. Cheaper, more delicious, and chemical-free, beans are not only easy to cook from scratch, they're practically mistake-proof. (You'll get the scoop in Part 2.)

Time to Take a Deep Breath

If this rather scary chapter has left you in such a state of dismay you wish you'd never picked up this book, let me remind you of two really cool things.

First, this hard-to-take information is followed by easy-to-use techniques and yummy recipes that will awaken exciting new tastebuds you never knew you had.

Second, I want to mention what leading health expert Dr. Dean Ornish calls the virtuous cycle—the higher levels of energy, mental clarity, and optimized health you'll feel after eliminating some of these common toxins from your diet. The rewards make it easier to adopt the changes, and once you've got them down, it's Beanalicious living all the way.

CHAPTER 9

Media on a Mission

Whoever said you can't be too rich or too thin apparently never watched reality TV. The past decade has proven that excess has its limits, from overspending to overusing to overeating; all these activities have consequences that are proving less than pleasant in the long term. We've been operating on overdrive for so long, we've come to accept that more is always better—without stopping to wonder, "When is enough . . . enough?"

Having spent quite a few years advocating for sustainable living, I also know how hard it is to evoke change, whether it's within ourselves or among others. But change is inevitable, as many of us are discovering, and it's not necessarily bad. Recent trends across the country are showcasing progressive concepts like the slow-food movement, which is based on practices once considered old-fashioned: growing your own, cooking from scratch, crafting by hand—many of the things our fast-paced society tossed aside in favor of expediency. But now it's time to pause for a moment, look around, and smell the beans. What have we given up in order to be able to have it ready to go, right now?

I'd like my three-bean chili without the cancer-causing chemicals, please. And I'd prefer not to pay more for processed foods when I can easily make them myself and create a healthier, tastier version while I'm at it. Oh, and by the way, you can hold the trans fats, chemicals, and corn syrup, too. Because in our haste to do more faster, we seem to have missed an important point.

What we eat matters to our health, the health of our bank accounts, and the health of the planet. When we began ignoring this fact in favor of the quick fix, we began to pay the price with epidemic levels of obesity on one hand, and rising rates of malnutrition among U.S. children on the other. It's hard to believe that this is happening right in our own backyards.

But the solutions exist, available and easier than you might think. When we vote with our dollars for foods requiring tremendous energy to grow, process, package, and ship, we're paying to allocate resources to more than just food-growing. We grow enough food in this country to provide every one of us with an ample supply of calories and nutrients. It's our deranged distribution system that's keeping some of us overfed and others hungry.

Industrial farming is big, bad, and centralized. With a mean combination of government subsidy money in one giant hand, and economies of scale on the other, Big Ag is able to write the menu for most of the U.S. by making the foods that bring them the most profit the most widely affordable and available.

Remember, though, that just because these industrial farmers can pump up their plants and animals with all sorts of concoctions to make them seem appealing *and* benefit from a regulatory system more dotted with loopholes than Swiss cheese, doesn't mean you have to buy their products. The meat industry, for example, has us so confused about animal protein that we're scared into submission. When I first moved to Santa Cruz, California, a progressive seaside community becoming as well-known for sustainable farming as for its spectacular surf, I was surprised by the number of vegetarians I encountered. More unusual still was the number of kids in my first-grader's class who didn't eat meat.

At the time I was quick to judge. "How hippy-dippy," I said to myself. "I'd *never* compromise my kids' health for my ideals. It's one thing to make those choices for yourself, but kids need their protein!"

A couple of years had to pass before it became clear to me that these vegetarian kids weren't lacking anything as far as I could see. They were just as likely to shine in the classroom and the soccer field as their meat-eating counterparts. I did some research then, and

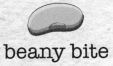

beany bite

Garbanzo beans are the top food source of vitamin B6, with just one cup containing 55% of the USDA recommended daily allowance.

learned that plant proteins are no compromise; in fact, the opposite is true, because eating nuts and beans in place of red meat or processed meat can lower the risk of heart disease and diabetes beginning in childhood.

Big Food companies will never admit that the natural healing properties abundant in so many whole foods are best left unprocessed, and that fortifying, supplementing, or adding extra nutrients compromises the outcome. A breakfast of steel-cut oatmeal, or a slice of sprouted wheat toast with almond milk and fruit, are much healthier choices than any processed cereal out there, no matter how much fiber and vitamins have been tossed in after the fact.

Why? Because the further away a food is processed from its natural state—like a flake of cereal without any recognizable original properties—the less efficacious its natural nutrients become, and no amount of last-minute supplementing will bring it up to par. Recently one evening, after a sumptuous dinner of white bean and collard green sauté, I sat down to check email. Scanning the list of subject lines, a promotion for a special new kidney-bean extract caught my eye. Apparently it's guaranteed to support weight loss and maintain healthy glucose levels.

The ironic part is that the fiber in whole foods such as beans, grains, and produce is a key component in a healthy diet, and the best way to get that is simply by eating the foods that provide it. How easy is that? So when USDA MyPlate guidelines say that it's okay to eat up to half of your daily allotment of grains via bread, cereal, rice, and pasta in their refined forms, I say: *hello empty carbs!* Stick with unprocessed plant foods for the whole, healthy nutrient package.

During digestion, refined grains, which have their fibrous properties removed, are converted to glucose immediately, just like sugar. Eating these foods can make it harder to control weight, and can raise the risk of heart disease and diabetes.

So why risk it? When making simple changes to your weekly meal plan can usher in a new dawn of well-being, let's kick it into gear and get those beans a-boiling!

A key point to keep in mind is that we haven't handed anything

beany bite

A US News & World Report health feature included beans among the top 8 sources of omega-3 fatty acids—polyunsaturated fats that play a crucial role in how our body's cells function.

over that we can't take back. Our relationship with Big Food isn't a partisan issue—it's a systemic problem. I see our governing system as a similar type of problem; it's broken and we know it, but rather than working to address it, the parties of power just keep pointing fingers.

But that doesn't make the food/health situation hopeless. Far from it. You and I can start by reclaiming our own power—right here, right now—by making a commitment to better health and all of the amazing benefits that go with it.

To quote one of my eco-heroes, Laurie David, the visionary environmental activist who produced Al Gore's groundbreaking *An Inconvenient Truth*: "We have to reject the trillion-dollar processed-food industry that's taken over our lives. Instead of buying salad dressing at the supermarket with 19 ingredients, we should be taking the three ingredients and the four minutes it takes to make salad dressings at home."

To which I say: Amen!

CHAPTER 10

Why Farms and Factories Just Don't Mix

Factory farming is the process of raising animals in highly confined, very crowded conditions. Since much of the business is automated and the animals are treated as product, this type of farm operates more like a factory than a home on the range.

While factory farms vary by animal type and region, the defining characteristic of a factory farm is that hundreds to thousands of animals (usually cows, pigs, chickens, or turkeys) are crowded tightly together and given little access to sunlight, fresh air, or even room to move. Some facilities "produce" millions of animals annually, raising obvious questions about how sustainable and ethical this practice is.

However, my intention isn't to proselytize animal rights. I want to focus on some of the reasons why factory-farmed products are downright unhealthy for people, too.

Most animals raised for food today come from factory farms. Unfortunately, the conditions at these establishments are so dirty that farmers have to resort to all kinds of questionable tactics to keep the animals from developing rampant disease, and to keep the animal products free from *E. coli* and other bacteria. In fact, 50% of antibiotics administered in the U.S. are used for animals, helping to create those creepy "superbugs" that are linked with serious illness and even death in humans.

Other practices are just as slimy. For example, after slaughter, factory-farmed chickens are washed in a chlorine bath containing 30 times more chlorine than the average swimming pool. To mask the smell and—according to chicken producers—to keep the meat moist while cooking, chickens are then injected with a solution of water and phosphate. Phosphate has been shown to increase the risk of chronic kidney disease, frail bones, and even premature aging. And to me, the very idea of chlorine-washed, phosphate-injected meat just sounds gross.

Beef fares no better. Factory-farmed cattle are routinely injected with hormones to help them grow faster and fatter, but it doesn't stop there. Keep in mind that you literally are what you eat; high-hormone foods impact human development in ways that still are not fully understood. Hormone residues in beef have been implicated in the early onset of puberty in girls, which could put them at greater risk of developing breast and other forms of cancer. And we do know that when runoff from factory farms enters nearby waterways, exposure to these growth hormones has a substantial effect on the gender and reproductive capacity of fish, disrupting natural growth cycles.

And if you happen to be concerned about toxins or pesticides, it's probably important to know that factory-farmed animal products, as in dairy and beef, contain more toxic residue than any farmed foods, since the chemicals are processed and stored in animal fat cells. For example, dioxin, a particularly potent chemical predominantly found in fatty meat and dairy products, is a toxin linked to lymphoma cancers in humans. Fabulous— why not just light up a Marlboro to enjoy with your burger?

So even when you're buying meat that says "USDA Prime" or "Grade A Ribeye" or any of the other impressive-sounding labels on factory-farmed meat, remember where it came from; 99% of the time it was straight from the factory.

By the way, I don't have a secret goal of driving you to veganism. But I believe you ought to know the facts about factory-farmed meat, and I hope to encourage you to consider the alternatives. And I know these facts can be disturbing—but not as unsettling as learning that through overexposure to antibiotics you've developed a resistance just at the time you really need them.

If you're like my daughter Hayden, who loves animals and understands unequivocally where meat comes from, yet still craves a burger now and then, grass-fed and free-range meat is the way to go. You may have a source in a local farm, or you can look for these designations stamped on packages in stores that carry natural foods. Raised in healthy, non-confined conditions, the products of these animals are chemical- and toxin-free, plus their production adds less pollution to the water and air, unlike that of their factory brethren. When in doubt, always ask, and if free-range costs more, you might try cutting back on meat in general for a win-win all around.

What about Factory-farmed Produce?

In the U.S., we're losing small, family-owned farms to industrial one-crop giants faster than you can say "Monoculture." Giant industrial plant-production facilities bring some shady practices to crop production that pollute the environment, and ultimately people, too. And as you may have guessed, switching the healthy variety of produce traditionally grown on a farm for a single, massive, monoculture crop that requires heavy chemical soil fertilization to keep producing isn't healthy for the soil, the environment, or the eater.

The next time you're at the grocery store, take a look at the fruits and vegetables. Ever wondered why they're so perfect-looking? Why they tend to be the same size, shape, and color? If it all seems a bit suspicious, then you're onto something. These monocrops are bred for longevity and their ability to ship well—the heck with flavor and nutrient levels. This is one trade-off I'd rather not make, thanks!

And then there's the pesticides. U.S. farmers use so much glyphosate, the main ingredient in weed killers like Roundup, that scientists are finding it in air, rain, and waterways. According to USDA figures, farmers sprayed 57 million pounds of glyphosate on food crops in 2009—mostly on genetically engineered soy and corn crops. Glyphosate is a systemic chemical, which means it works its way into the plants; since 85% of commercially grown soy and corn is fed to animals, it ultimately ends up on our plates. This chemical is linked to both diet-related disease and developmental disorders.

beany bite

Beans are good for the planet! According to the Environmental Working Group's "Meat Eater's Guide," lentils top the list of climate-friendly protein sources.

In fact, lots of the chemicals used to grow non-organic food are toxins. They include hormone disruptors, which scientists are starting to discover tamper with our body's natural weight-management abilities. Some pesticides are linked to obesity, and others are linked in a growing number of studies with diabetes. While results are inconclusive at present, especially regarding the levels and types of exposure, I believe it makes sense to go organic when you can. For a lot of us, the word "organic" is synonymous with "expensive," and it may not be affordable or even available. But where you can, it's worth it. Farmers' markets, farm stands, and farm co-ops are great places to find pesticide-free or organic products.

And some produce retains more pesticide residue than others. When you can't do it all, here's a list of the top 12 fruits and vegetables to try to buy organic, courtesy of the Environmental Working Group:

1. Apples
2. Celery
3. Sweet bell peppers
4. Peaches
5. Strawberries
6. Nectarines
7. Grapes
8. Spinach
9. Lettuce
10. Cucumbers
11. Blueberries
12. Potatoes

Shopping locally and eating in season keeps this more manageable. Knowing the facts and doing your best are a strong first step.

Marketing Thin at the Expense of Healthy
In-the-package and on-the-go have replaced healthy whole foods for too many of us. We don't have time to cook, we don't know how, or the thought of slaving over a stove makes our hair stand on end. We're already so overbooked that cooking from scratch just isn't an

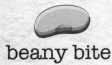

beany bite

Harvard School of Public Health researchers concluded that women who consume beans at least twice per week are 24% less likely to develop breast cancer than non–bean-eaters.

option, and a girl's got to eat (low-fat foods, of course)!

Since the time we're old enough to notice, Americans are constantly bombarded with messages telling us how happy a perfect appearance will make us. The ironic thing is that most of the time these messages are coming from people trying to sell us either food or weight-loss products. I've said it before and I'll say it again: the best dietary choices—the most naturally nutritious, delicious, and low in saturated fat—don't come in a package. Processed food never trumps fresh. The nutrients and ingredients used to "fortify" processed food originate from fresh, whole foods, where they belong.

But since processed-food companies sell, yes, processed food, and they have millions of dollars to tell us why we need it, that's what they pitch. Ads showing super-fit young women in bikinis looking amazing because they ate the special breakfast bar don't just sound too good to be true, they are. Newsflash: it wasn't the breakfast bar that makes her look like that and, by the way, I'd like to see her kitchen cabinets. The likelihood they're stocked with processed foods? Slim to none!

Humans are hard-wired with a need to fit in, and we'll sometimes do anything to get there. Those extra pounds can creep up unnoticed, until we suddenly find ourselves self-conscious and uncomfortable. Which is how they getcha. Suddenly the situation seems critical, because all too often it happens the week before the event you need to squeeze into that little black dress for.

Driven to desperation, you frantically flip through this month's *In Style* for a solution. You choose from among a bevy of so-called cures, landing on the most simple and straightforward. Grapefruit and diet pills for a week? No problem! In the end you lose the weight, and look the part, but when the methods are unhealthy, even a perfect size 6 is not going to make you happy. Plus, you're so hungry by the time that diet is over, you nosh your way up a size just trying to feel normal again.

Unfortunately, these misguided diet patterns often take root in adolescence, when we tend to be most vulnerable. I was among these classic American teens. Once I hit puberty, poor eating habits and lack of exercise brought on the excess pounds—and all the social issues

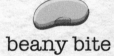

beany bite

Legumes are a good source of folate (also known as folic acid), the B vitamin essential for normal brain function. Recent Mayo Clinic research links low levels of folate with Alzheimer's disease.

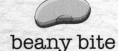

beany bite

Beans as a symbol of fertility? Yes! In ancient Rome, black beans were believed to be so potent that nuns were banned from eating them; it was feared that the beans would seduce them into betraying their vows of chastity.

that come with it. There was no denying I was chubby, a condition I soon learned that for high school girls was simply not acceptable. Fortunately we savvy teens had access to a slew of helpful products to help make us look like the people in the magazines. There were diet pills, diet drinks, fad diets, starvation, and, when all else failed, eating disorders.

I lost the excess weight, but I suffered for it. My poor diet left me unhappy, unhealthy, and unfocused. It took many, many years of trial and error, studying the effects of diet on my personal health along with in-depth research into numerous expert nutritional findings, to discover a better way.

And I love what I've discovered: that healthy eating simply means getting back to the basics of whole, unprocessed, chemical-free food. No more diets, no more deprivation. Just luscious, whole-foods living.

CHAPTER 11

To Meat or Not to Meat?

Meat is one of those subjects best broached lightly. It tends to heat up a conversation really fast and I've got to admit I've touched a few hot spots here and there. In this country, we love us some brisket! Holidays, sporting events, Lady Gaga—so many things in our culture are associated with meat, and second-guessing them is a task not lightly undertaken.

Nonetheless, I'm going out on a limb here and doing it anyway. There's way too much shady stuff going on behind the scenes; I think you should know what it is you're really dealing with. The good news is, there's no pressure to hop aboard the Tofu Express if your goal is better health. Reducing your meat consumption can be a process like any other, and the good news is, there are plenty of enticing alternatives to Tofurky.

While my focus in *Beanalicious Living* is on healthy eating, not climate change, it would be remiss not to mention that according to a United Nations report, the meat industry produces more greenhouse gases than the world's plane, train, and automobile fleets combined. The livestock sector (i.e., factory farms) is the leading contributor to water pollution in the U.S., thanks to nitrogen and phosphorus runoff. A third of all U.S. fuel consumption is attributed to livestock production.

Meanwhile, back on the nutrition front: big news came recently with findings from a major study from Harvard University on meat and mortality. Researchers followed more than 100,000 men and women—and their diets—for up to 22 years. They found that red meat consumption was associated with "living a significantly shorter life as a result of increased cancer mortality, increased heart disease mortality, and increased overall mortality." Any sentence containing the word "mortality" three times certainly sounds bad, but what does it mean?

Leading health expert Dr. Joel Fuhrman summarizes it simply: "The [Harvard study] authors concluded each daily serving of unprocessed red meat increased [mortality] risk by 13% and processed meat by 20%. However, the bottom line 'red meat increases risk of mortality' certainly isn't news."

Now, don't panic. This study didn't differentiate between grass-fed and factory-farmed meats, and as I explained in gory detail in Chapter 10, factory farming is a key health-risk factor in meat consumption.

For many of us, meat is an important part of our diet. At the same time, the scientific evidence is increasingly clear that eating too much meat—particularly red and processed meat—is associated with a wide variety of serious health problems. But the good news for carnivores is that not all meat is created equal. Grass-fed meat and dairy have been identified in a number of studies as an important source of certain nutrients.

According to authors Tyler Graham and Dr. Drew Ramsey in their book *The Happiness Diet,* meat isn't the problem, factory-farmed meat is. Their research shows that of the 588 different combinations of fats found within the human profile, some are good and some are bad, but mostly we don't yet know enough to make specific, scientifically based recommendations. However, we do know a few fat facts for certain.

Trans fats from hydrogenated vegetable oils are bad for us. Conjugated linoleic acid (CLA), derived only from meat and animal products, specifically grass-fed ruminants such as cows, is very good for us. Graham and Ramsey contend that CLA increases blood flow to the brain, protects brain-cell longevity, and counteracts the effects of the stress hormone cortisol. And grass-fed meats routinely show higher levels of omega-3 fatty acids and other vitamins, as well as lower levels of *E. coli*, than factory-farmed beef.

I haven't eaten red meat in 25 years, so does this mean most of my life's stress could have been prevented with a daily dose of liverwurst? As it turns out, the most concentrated sources are found in milk and cheese, especially goat and sheep's milk. CLA is said to prevent some cancers, promote muscle growth, and prevent abdominal fat deposits. In that case, bring on the goat cheese! But meat?

I believe that responsibly farmed and harvested meat or seafood eaten in moderation can be a good source of complete protein and key nutrients such as iron, zinc, vitamin B12, vitamin B6, and niacin (although experts remind us that plants adequately provide all except B12 as well). One thing is certain, though: as a nation we eat too few vegetables and too much meat.

Americans eat more meat than most other developed nations, almost more than all the rest combined. In 2009, the U.S. produced 208 pounds of meat per person for domestic consumption, not including seafood. That's nearly 60% more than Europe produced and nearly four times as much as most developing countries.

Recent research suggests that eating all this meat is contributing to the U.S. obesity epidemic. It's no surprise that several major studies have found an association between high meat-consumption levels and being overweight, but did you know it's actually been quantified? A 2009 Johns Hopkins University study found that regular meat-eaters (as in standard portions eaten at most meals, every day) ate an average of 700 calories more per day and, other factors being equal, had a 27% greater likelihood of being obese than meat-eaters who consumed the least.

A similar European study found that men and women who ate the most meat consumed an average of 900 and 600 more calories per day, respectively, than those who ate the least. The study attributed weight gain to the high fat content and calories in many meats and concluded that "a decrease in meat consumption may improve weight management," which just makes sense since meat doesn't contain the filling fiber and satisfying nutrients of plant proteins. Dr. Dean Ornish points out that the body recognizes the volume of food ingested as a sign of satiety, so fiber-rich foods are the way to go for weight management.

But even if you're happy with your weight, and these findings are

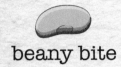

beany bite

a non-issue for you, a more common meat-eater's concern is the P word: protein. I regularly visit a vegetarian retreat center whose main attraction is yoga. Most of the yoga devotees aren't vegetarians and they express a lot of concern about their diet during a two-day visit. Will they be getting enough protein, they worry, from the center's meat-free cuisine?

So let me share with you some simple stats. In the U.S., 16–18% of our calories come from protein. The average daily recommended allowance is 10%. I'm no mathematician, but it's easy to see we're exceeding that by 60–80%. Now—stay with me here—80% of this protein we're consuming comes from animal products. When we compare this to nations with far lower consumption-related disease rates such as rural China (which has about a 10% rate of animal-based protein consumption), it turns out to be almost 10 times more. Yes, there *is* a connection. Too much animal protein leads to diet-related diseases such as obesity, high cholesterol, heart disease, and cancer. Extensive research proves this.

The good news is that despite what most people believe, protein is found in more than just meat. In fact, studies show it would be difficult *not* to get enough protein if you're eating a healthy, plant-based diet.

As mentioned above, protein intake for most age groups far exceeds our own government's recommended dietary allowance, which is by many considered quite generous. By contrast, only 1% of children and 4% of adults eat their recommended daily intake of fruits and vegetables. Holy guacamole! Any way you slice it, we're eating too much meat, too much protein, and way too few fruits and vegetables.

I know most meat lovers aren't going to give up the goat entirely, but there are lots of great reasons to bring some alternative proteins into our diet. A number of studies have found that people who eat vegetarian diets have lower rates of chronic disease and often live longer than those on predominantly meat-based diets. The American Dietetic Association, the world's largest organization of nutrition experts, maintains that vegetarians have less obesity and lower rates of chronic medical conditions such as heart disease, diabetes, and hypertension.

Scientific evidence is making it increasingly clear that eating too much meat, particularly factory-farmed and processed meat, is associated with a wide variety of serious health problems. Leading healthcare expert Dr. Joseph Mercola strongly recommends avoiding factory-farmed meat; it is, he says, "significantly inferior in quality and nutrition, and the harm will likely outweigh the benefits for most people."

While we're on the topic, I'd like to clarify a common (and possibly intentionally cultivated) misconception. Chicken is still meat, and despite what pork producers have tried to convince us, white is not necessarily a health benefit. Tests of chicken samples from large-scale poultry producers have shown traces of a number of pharmaceuticals, including active ingredients used in Benadryl, Tylenol, and Prozac, as well as residues of fluoroquinolone antibiotics, drugs which were banned from poultry production since 2005. It's one thing to find these products in your medicine chest, and much as I'm sometimes tempted to turn to Prozac, I'd prefer not to have it delivered in my chicken.

On Following a "Diet"

While diet trends generally focus on specific food groups, then strictly enforce their inclusion or dismissal, the rate of success stays despairingly low. But rather than demonizing an entire whole-foods group as in carbs, fats, or even sustainably produced animal products, maybe it's time to reframe the argument. I appreciate *New York Times* columnist and author Mark Bittman's astute observation on the universal conundrum of meat versus vegetable in his book *How to Cook Everything*. Bittman forecasts a trend toward reduced meat consumption—if not for health reasons, then economic ones. Simply put, he suggests our current way of eating is not long-term sustainable.

If Bittman's forecast rings in a tad dreary, you'll be happy to hear the rest. He explains: "Increasingly, Americans are becoming 'flexitarians,' a recently invented word that describes vegetarians that aren't that strict and meat-eaters that are striving for a more health-conscious, planet-friendly diet." Meat is just too resource-heavy; for example, it's

beany bite

Certain bean types are used in Chinese medicine to treat diseases such as high blood pressure, kidney stones, rheumatism, and dozens of other conditions.

estimated that it takes 2,500 gallons of water to produce a single pound of beef. Or as *Newsweek* magazine puts it: "The water that goes into a 1,000-pound steer would float a destroyer." Add to that the land-use requirements, increased carbon emissions, and other waste-disposal issues; it's my belief that our current level of consumption needs rethinking. Luckily we have other options which are much more adaptive.

Ready to Cut Down On—Or Cut Out—the Meat?

Does the thought of eliminating meat from your diet leave you weak in the knees? If so, don't fret; it needn't be so black and white. If you can't (or don't want to) quit, start by reducing the amount you eat—one meal a day if you can. But even just one day a week makes a difference. Hipster mamas like Drew Barrymore, Jessica Simpson, and Gywneth Paltrow are part of the Meat Free Monday movement, a fun and visionary theme you can bring into your life. My kids are into it, and Neal, who would eat meat every Monday if he did the shopping, proudly sports his Meat Free Monday tee anyway. (I bought it for him, of course!)

Does this sound a bit daunting? I know how hard it is to make changes. Because I live this stuff, knowing all I know about factory farms has made it easier for me to go veg. But Neal? That's a whole 'nother story. He knows the facts, too—I remind him more often than he would like (while trying to stay subtle, lest he tune me out entirely)— yet at a restaurant he'll still blithely order the factory-farmed chicken burrito over the veggie option. But when I cook, which is most of the time, he doesn't miss the animal protein, because the plant-based, high-protein bean and grain dishes are so delicious and satisfying.

So if you're ready to give it a go, find the strategy that works for you, whether it's all at once or, as I mentioned in Chapter 3, "leaning into it," a little at a time. Not sure where to start? Meat Free Monday is a perfect first step toward healthier living, maybe even a fun family ritual; it can open the door to new ways of cooking. Not harder, maybe easier—just fresh and more creative.

There are tons of easy recipes to experiment with that are so tasty

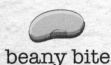

beany bite

The USDA recommends eating at least 3 cups of beans each week for optimal nutritional benefits, which is three times more than the current weekly average.

and satiating the meat won't even be missed. The recipes featured in *Beanalicious Living* are an easy and delicious way to start. The internet is another great resource for recipes, as are libraries and bookstores for inspiring cookbooks. I love to cook this way and often serve meat-free dinners to nonvegetarian friends, most of whom are happy to be introduced to vegetarian cooking, sometimes for the first time. They're frequently pleasantly surprised by my meaty portobello mushrooms, tasty lentils, and hearty vegetarian chili.

When you start feeling better after upgrading your diet with power-packed, plant-based protein, meat-free might just start expanding out to the rest of your week.

There's another benefit, too, for those of us with families. This kind of dietary exploration easily expands into a new topic of conversation with kids. How do our personal choices impact the world around us and even affect our future? I'm not sure how often this gets discussed in our schools, so it's all the more important for it to be discussed at home.

I've been up-front with my kids from day one. I don't eat meat because of the inhumane way animals are treated, and because I don't believe it's good for me. Other people have different opinions, I've explained, but those are my reasons for promoting a plant-based diet in our family. That said, I leave my girls free to make their own choices when appropriate; I just try to steer things away from factory farming.

Hayden seems to crave meat, so I'd offer her a grass-fed burger every now and then. One day, we were heading home from the beach when she suddenly announced she was a vegetarian.

"Great!" I responded, wondering how this sudden change of heart had come about.

"Look!" she said to Talia, pointing to something I couldn't see since they were in the back and I was driving. "It's a baby cow. I don't want to eat *that!*"

Talia gasped. "I'm a vegetarian, too!" she exclaimed.

"Fantastic!" was my short, yet enthusiastic response.

Since the day of declaration, Hayden has occasionally enjoyed some free-range chicken nuggets, but she's making a conscious choice,

beany bite

Beans have staying power. A Brigham Young University study tested beans stored for up to 32 years. A consumer panel gave them an 80% approval rating for taste appeal.

not an industry-manufactured one. And as for Talia, she never ate meat anyway so I guess she was just making it official.

As adults, it really comes down to discovering for yourself whether a meat-free diet changes the way your body feels. Most people experience weight loss and increased energy; additionally, studies show that overall health generally improves long-term with reduced meat intake.

I know this first-hand. Neal was diagnosed with high blood pressure, a condition closely related to heart disease. He was put on two different medications and experienced some unpleasant side effects, including passing out randomly more than once. It was scary enough that I began to wonder which was worse, the sickness or the treatment. It was pure coincidence that we began seriously revamping our diet around that time, more due to environmental motivation than for health concerns. I won't say Neal was (or is) on board with plant-based eating all the time, but since I do the shopping and cooking, he's pretty much stuck.

Fast forward to several years later, and Neal has become a whole new person. His tastes have changed, his weight has dropped, and he says he'll never go back to his former lifestyle. Since he's reduced his meat consumption dramatically and switched to grass-fed when he *does* partake at home, he's ditched the meds and found good health again. Now I know anything is possible!

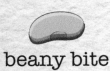

beany bite

In the South, eating black-eyed peas and greens (such as collards) on New Year's Day is considered good luck: the beans symbolize coins and the greens symbolize paper money.

Top 10 Reasons to Eat Less Meat

1. Debunk the protein myth. Rethink your vision of the anemic vegetarian: some of the strongest animals on earth are plant-eaters, and some of the strongest people, like Carl Lewis and Martina Navratilova, are, too! (Not to mention other fascinating vegetarians such as Ellen DeGeneres, Fred Rogers, Natalie Portman, Cesar Chávez, George Barnard Shaw, Leonardo da Vinci, Thomas Alva Edison, Albert Einstein, Jane Goodall, Rosa Parks, Russell Simmons, and Sir Paul McCartney!)

2. Reduce your risk of some major diseases. Meat and meat products are linked to a variety of health problems. And, according to the American Dietetic Association, "a vegetarian diet may provide health benefits in the prevention and treatment of certain diseases."

3. Keep your eye on the bottom line. Pound for pound, legumes and vegetables deliver more nutritional value for less money.

4. Do it for the planet. If everyone in the U.S. ate no meat or cheese just one day a week, it would be like not driving 91 billion miles—or taking 7.6 million cars off the road.

5. You'll feel better, since aligning your eating habits more closely with even the most conservative dietary recommendations will lead to a healthier you. A 2010 American Society for Nutrition report shows that 98% of us are missing the mark for legumes and whole grains while we're surpassing most recommendations for meat and dairy consumption. Swap your way to better health and you'll be pleasantly surprised when you feel the rejuvenating results.

6. And speaking of rejuvenation, you'll look better, too!

7. Enjoy the opportunity to discover a veritable plethora of fresh produce. Whether you grow your own food or sprout your own seeds, or frequent farmers' markets, farm stands, or your local produce market, let your inner chef go wild!

8. You'll stop contributing to damaging farming conditions. Unless explicitly noted, most livestock raised for food live on factory farms, which are not only dreadful places for animals, they're highly polluting.

9. You'll avoid antibiotics, hormones, and other synthetic chemicals which are administered to factory-farmed animals to make them grow fatter faster and stay infection-free in dirty, crowded conditions.

10. You'll discover a whole new world of delicious cuisine. And don't worry if you're not a kitchen ninja—*Beanalicious Living* serves up everything you need to cook healthy, eat well, and still have a life.

CHAPTER 12

Nutrition Label Shakedown

In Part 2, the Beanalicious simple menu and planning guide will help make home-cooked a healthy habit that's easy to keep, even if cooking is less than your favorite activity. In that case, chances are you won't be making everything from scratch. Much as I love homemade salsa, snacks, and sauces, there are lots of times when healthy, pre-made foods are an absolute lifesaver (as in almost every day).

The good news is, you don't have to choose between easy and healthy—you can have both. In the preceding chapters, I've talked about how to identify the biggest processed-food culprits. Now let's take a closer look at how to avoid them.

Step into any grocery store and you'll see lots of products which make enticing claims like "Whole-grain," "Healthy," "All-natural," "Organic," and "Trans-fat Free." As I've touched on elsewhere in this book, choosing foods based on the glossy pictures and glorious promises on the front of the package is like getting your facts from the *National Enquirer.* Not always so reliable.

In fact, many of the so-called "health foods" contain some of the worst ingredients. Because who decides whether or not it's a health food? Yep—the manufacturer! Remember Jeff Novick from Chapter 7? He's a former Kraft Foods executive turned nutritionist and healthy-diet spokesperson and he bluntly summarizes it like this: "Don't believe what you read on the front label—*ever!*" According to Novick, a recent Cornell poll found that more than 84% of American shoppers are confused about their nutrition choices. I guess those labels aren't helping.

Food labels are confusing by design. It's easy to make unsubstan-tiated health claims on the front of the package, and easier still if the Nutrition Facts on the side make no sense. For example, where you see the number of grams of fat per serving listed on the package, they're actually calculated by weight, not as a percentage of the product you're purchasing. Consequently, 1% milk contains 25% fat; the fat just weighs 1% per serving.

Make sense? I didn't think so.

Food labels are not only confusing, they're tiny! But reading them is important, because when you must eat processed (and at least some of the time, most of us must) you don't have to eat junk. By making it hard to read and understand the information, manufacturers give themselves plenty of latitude when it comes to ingredients. So even if you can barely make out the words, take the time and do the legwork to source your goods. You'll be able to navigate the grocery store aisles more easily once you know what to look for.

Fortunately for us, the savvy Mr. Novick has boiled things down to some simple rules of thumb so if you have to buy packaged foods, at least there's less of a risk factor. Keep in mind Novick's most incon-venient truth and rule #1: *never* believe the claims on the front of the package.

Here are some tips for healthier food selection

· For most of us, trying to avoid sugar is like avoiding sun exposure. We know we should, but it's everywhere and it's so much fun. But when on average we consume five times the daily recommended allowance of added sugars, limiting is a good idea. Avoid products containing sugar of any kind in the first five ingredients and you're on the right track.

· Sodium content should never exceed the number of calories; look for a 1:1 ratio. If a serving of Pop Chips contains 100 calories, be sure it also contains less than 100 grams of sodium. Simple!

· Shift your focus from fat grams per serving, since serving sizes are quite subjective. Fat content should be no more than 20% of the total calorie content and should contain no trans fats. How to tell? Read the Nutrition Label on the back of the package, find the total calories per serving, and divide by 5. If fat calories are more than 20% of total calories, or if it contains hydrogenated anything, put it back.

More labeling tricks to look out for

- Make sure you're buying whole grains. Claims announcing "Whole-wheat" or "Multi-grain" on the front are not the same thing. Read the Nutrition Label carefully to make sure the word "whole" precedes every grain listed, or look for the "100% whole-grain" claim. This is one term regulated by the FDA to ensure that all grains used in the product are, in fact, whole.

- Beware of serving sizes. Not all serving sizes are the same, nor do they necessarily make sense. That individually wrapped granola bar may proudly announce only 50 calories per serving, but you'd have to scrutinize the fine print to discover there are really three servings per bar.

- Beware of words you don't know or recognize in the ingredients. If you wouldn't stock them in your kitchen, it's because they don't belong in your food!

- Avoid products containing sodium nitrate, a preservative that's commonly used in processed meats like bacon, jerky, and lunch meats. Studies link nitrates to diabetes and heart disease.

- Beware of hidden sugars in processed foods. The most common tactic to keep sugar from the top of the ingredients list? Mixing the names of different sweeteners so the weight is spread out among several forms of sugar. The ones to look out for: honey, dextrose, corn syrup, high-fructose corn syrup, maple syrup, molasses, sucrose, fructose, maltose, and lactose.

Unfortunately for us, manufacturers often take a perfectly healthy food item, put it in a box, toss in some unnecessary additives, and market it as the newest, hottest health-food star. Case in point: I recently spotted a box of "Easy Quinoa" at the natural-foods store where I shop. To me, "easy" quinoa in a box makes as much sense as buying your food pre-chewed. It's just bulk quinoa, placed in a package decked out with alluring pictures on the front, all designed to entice you to pay more.

Manufacturers are highly proficient at spotting food trends. Any new food item that scores some press—whether for nutritional value, taste, or simple novelty—becomes a hot target for all kinds of new products

Meanwhile the practice of stripping the nutrients out of whole foods through processing, than adding them back in, often in synthetic versions, is still in question. When you live the Beanalicious lifestyle, you'll enjoy healthy, satisfying whole foods simply prepared to retain flavor and nutritional value—no guesswork required.

Cooking rice and grains is not rocket science. If you can boil water, you can cook quinoa. But by adding a few seasonings and putting it into a box with a fancy name and some snazzy proclamations, like "Easy," "Healthy," and "Gluten-free," something that should be pretty basic suddenly sounds like you'd better buy it packaged, just in case. Heck, why not just add these kinds of descriptions to a bottle of plain old water? Oh, right—that's been done.

But back to this "Easy Quinoa" business. Now that we've established that the bulk bin or unadulterated pre-packed quinoa is just as easy, what else do you get for that extra cash? Typically some dubious additions like potato starch, sugar, and 10 times the recommended level of sodium. Just one more reminder that words like "Natural" and "Healthy" are just marketing-speak. Always, always, read the label to get the facts.

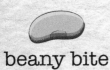

beany bite

According to David Grotto, R.D., author of 101 Foods That Could Save Your Life, black beans have been shown to block the circulation of estradiol, a form of estrogen linked to breast cancer.

CHAPTER 13

Cooking from
(Dare I Say?)
Scratch

So is this book just about beans? Of course not. It's about taking steps toward better health, more energy, and a slimmer you in ways that are sustainable—and manageable long-term. In order to make change, you need options you can embrace. As in more fun, less tedium.

Cooking with beans will bring out your culinary creativity because they're so easy, inexpensive, and versatile. We all enjoy good home cooking: the fresh flavors, the healthy preparation, the palatable price tag. We just don't necessarily know how, or want to take the time to do it. Figuring out menus, buying a lot of different ingredients which you aren't necessarily familiar with, maybe having to purchase in large quantities when you only need a little, then learning how to prepare the dish—it's a lot of work and may not be your first-choice way to spend what little "extra" time you have.

Since free time is a luxury few of us have enough of, we need a bold new style of simple cooking and meal preparation to get us through. The beauty of beans is that once you know the basics, you can devise and customize salads, dips, and side-dish recipes quite easily, just by incorporating the fresh ingredients you like. Beans store really well once cooked, so the trick is to prepare a multi-dish quantity two or three times a week, then work them into salads, sautés, soups, stews, or side dishes as much as your time and motivation permit.

An achievable starting goal is to substitute beans for a prepackaged restaurant meal or processed option you're currently eating.

Maybe you can begin with switching one meal a day. For example, if you have an energy bar for breakfast each day, try replacing it with a Beanalicious enzyme-rich green smoothie. Or instead of the mac and cheese you planned to enjoy with your hot dog for dinner, whip up some delicious Caribbean Black Beans. Or you could try switching your Subway salad for a homemade, super-healthy

White Bean Caesar Salad, and use the time you save standing in line to take a walk after lunch. (You'll find these three recipes in Part 2.)

It's my belief that we are better off by opting out of the processed/prepackaged system and supporting local food choices to the best of our ability. It's not about being perfect. If you think that without a 100% commitment you're a failure, you might be too daunted to even take those first steps. As the old saying goes, "Perfect is the enemy of the good." Just *trying* is more than okay in my book.

For a lot of us, home cooking is a challenging prospect. Assuming you eat three meals a day, that's 21 meals a week that you need to plan, shop for, and make. That sounds like the equivalent of taking a second (unpaid) job—unless, of course, you have some guidelines, tips, and suggestions for making the most of your time in the kitchen, which is where *Beanalicious Living* can help. In effect, the Beanalicious eating plan is about maximizing nutrients while minimizing the harder things like cost, calories, and preparation time. Beans can make all this a lot easier.

Most recipes revolve around a star ingredient and/or a flavor profile. But when I cook bean, grain, or vegetable dishes, I don't usually follow recipes—most of which are complicated and too time-consuming. Instead I work with themes, I know cooking times and techniques, and I use what I have available in my kitchen. "Which is all well and fine," you may be thinking, "but how does that help *me?*"

As part of my Beanalicious education and research, I recognized that while I now find cooking from scratch easy and approachable, not everyone feels this way, and I wanted to understand why. I'm not especially organized, I've never been to cooking school, but I like to cook. What was I doing differently that makes it more enjoyable?

I realized that in order to make home cooking manageable in my own life, I had begun working more recipes around my star ingredient, which was beans. One pot of beans yields countless versions of soup, dips, salads, and burritos. I started keeping five or six varieties in my pantry. With a batch or two of cooked beans in the fridge, in one week I could quickly whip up—for example—Beanalicious Garbanzo Bean Salad, House Blend Hummus, Minestrone Soup, and Curried Chickpeas and Potatoes. (And yes, you'll find these scrumptious recipes in Part 2.)

Now, what about "flavor profile"? This refers to the style of cuisine, as in Mexican, Thai, Italian, and so on. A dish can be prepared using signature requisites like pepper, onion, tomato, and cilantro for an enticing Mexican flair. Or you may decide to Thai one on with basil, chili peppers, and peanuts for a completely different flavor experience. Once you learn which ingredients work together and approximate ratios to use, the rest is easy.

Think of the salad bar at your favorite market or restaurant. You choose your main ingredient, usually greens, then add an assortment of your favorite shredded and cooked vegetables, a few toppings, maybe some seasoning, and finally dressing. *Voilà!* You've created a tasty salad without giving it a second thought. Now imagine the greens are replaced with cooked garbanzo beans. You add chopped tomato, cucumber, olives, and feta cheese, top it with olive oil, balsamic vinegar, and some seasonings, and you've created a Mediterranean salad worthy of five-star Epicurious.com ratings.

You can do this just as easily with the dishes you prepare at home. It's all about learning which ingredients work together, how to prepare things in advance, and knowing what you can safely buy pre-made (but not processed) to keep your meals simple to make and delicious to eat. Changing your eating habits is a big undertaking, and planning ahead is essential.

As willpower expert and author Dr. Kelly McGonigal explains, we make an average of 227 food-related choices in *just one day*. Most of these choices are made without much consideration. We're busy in our lives, distracted with other things, and not overly interested in

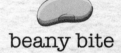

beany bite

Beans are a rich source of zinc, a mineral necessary for strengthening the immune system to protect against illness.

scrutinizing ingredients to determine which granola bar doesn't contain the exact same ingredients as an oatmeal cookie. We typically just grab and go.

This is where planning ahead is critical. You now know the reasons to make the switch from the easy, habit-entrenched foods that are not so good for you to fresh and healthy whole foods, but changing these habits often takes more than one "aha" moment. Changing your eating habits is a transition with a learning curve, meaning it may not happen all at once. And that's okay.

When you get to Part 2, "The Beanalicious Solution: Preparation Guide and Recipes," I invite you to familiarize yourself with the techniques, tips, and recipes, and decide what works for you. If you know there's just no way you're going to start off preparing all of your meals at home, celebrate the changes you *can* commit to . . . and add on from there. Doing what feels manageable will increase your long-term odds of success, so make it work for you.

If you're short on inspiration, let me share this story as told by one of the world's foremost authorities on diet and nutrition, Dr. Dean Ornish. During the Clinton Administration, Dr. Ornish was invited by Mrs. Clinton to act as nutritional consultant to the First Family, a position he holds to this day with the Clintons. Passionate as he is about the benefits of a whole-foods, plant-based diet, which his life's research and teachings support, he gladly accepted. During that time, President Clinton was suffering from pretty serious heart disease, in spite of a previous bypass.

The prez evidently experienced some health improvements by adopting some of Ornish's suggestions, but reportedly was still a fast-food lover and frequent customer. "It's the genes" a lot of doctors insisted. But in 2005, when his bypass failed and his health was rapidly deteriorating, Clinton was ready to give the Ornish program another try. Dr. Ornish and Dr. Caldwell Esselstyn, another leading diet and nutrition expert, advised Clinton to step up and take control of his health destiny, starting with diet.

Upon discovering that 82% of people who adopt Ornish's recommendations experience a reversal of chronic, diet-related disease, a newly motivated Clinton dove in. The results were nothing short of dramatic. And in May 2012, Clinton, also a former "milk mustache" model, began Dr. Esselstyn's diet program, which has been proven effective in reversing heart disease in 100% of people who stick to it. A few months later and many pounds lighter, he looks and reports feeling wonderful. And Clinton mentions beans as one of his new diet staples in a CNN interview! Overall, the diet is pretty straightforward: skip the meat, hold the dairy, and bring on the plant-based whole foods. Now, we know first-hand that even presidents don't always have perfect self-control, so I'm guessing if Bill Clinton can do it, so can you and I!

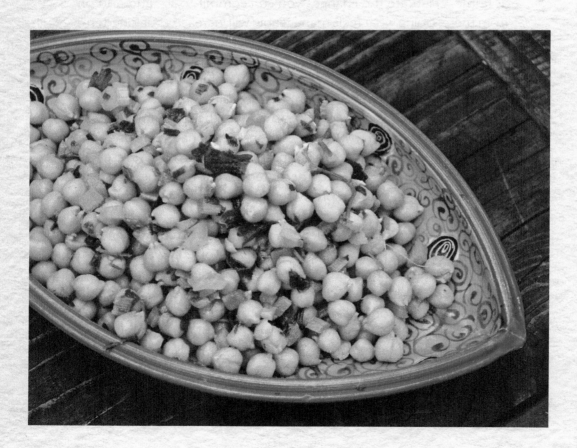

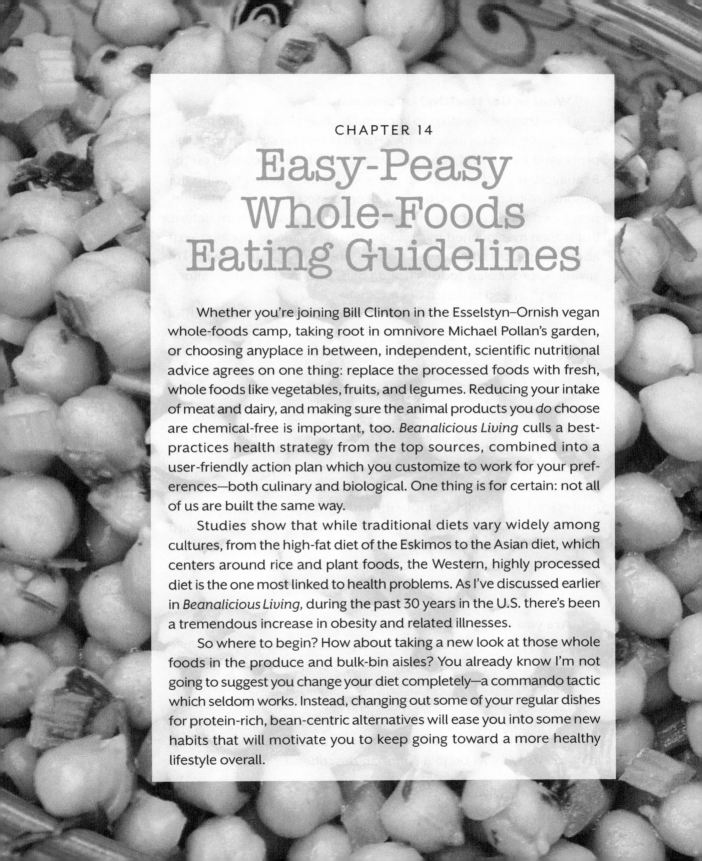

CHAPTER 14

Easy-Peasy Whole-Foods Eating Guidelines

Whether you're joining Bill Clinton in the Esselstyn–Ornish vegan whole-foods camp, taking root in omnivore Michael Pollan's garden, or choosing anyplace in between, independent, scientific nutritional advice agrees on one thing: replace the processed foods with fresh, whole foods like vegetables, fruits, and legumes. Reducing your intake of meat and dairy, and making sure the animal products you *do* choose are chemical-free is important, too. *Beanalicious Living* culls a best-practices health strategy from the top sources, combined into a user-friendly action plan which you customize to work for your preferences—both culinary and biological. One thing is for certain: not all of us are built the same way.

Studies show that while traditional diets vary widely among cultures, from the high-fat diet of the Eskimos to the Asian diet, which centers around rice and plant foods, the Western, highly processed diet is the one most linked to health problems. As I've discussed earlier in *Beanalicious Living,* during the past 30 years in the U.S. there's been a tremendous increase in obesity and related illnesses.

So where to begin? How about taking a new look at those whole foods in the produce and bulk-bin aisles? You already know I'm not going to suggest you change your diet completely—a commando tactic which seldom works. Instead, changing out some of your regular dishes for protein-rich, bean-centric alternatives will ease you into some new habits that will motivate you to keep going toward a more healthy lifestyle overall.

Want to Get Healthy? Unprocess!

Now that we've gotten to know each other after all these pages, I have a confession to make. Ready? Here it is: I eat certain commercially processed foods. And you know what? In all likelihood, even on the Beanalicious lifestyle plan, so will you. Whole-grain wheat bread, almond milk, coconut oil, tofu . . . all processed foods. By definition, processed food can be anything that originally comes from nature, but is then manipulated by grinding, blending, juicing, cooking—just about any process that takes it from its whole-food state. So what I'm saying is, processed food is not *all* bad, but it's the highly refined versions you need to watch out for.

Refined foods are stripped of some of their most healthful elements, as in whole grains in which the bran or germ is removed, leaving a nutritionally devoid product like white bread or rice. Go for whole over processed when you can, and for all the times you can't bake your own whole-wheat bread or whip up your own almond milk, I suggest you take a moment to read those labels carefully.

The *Beanalicious Living* meal-planning strategy combines common themes from the most well-respected wellness researchers, nutritionists, and healthy-eating organizations on the planet. I've based my recommendations on the work of best-selling author and Cornell professor Dr. T. Colin Campbell; leading dietary experts Dr. Joel Fuhrman, Dr. Caldwell Esselstyn, and Dr. Dean Ornish; the Harvard Medical School's Division of Nutrition, the Center for Science in the Public Interest, the Physicians Committee for Responsible Medicine, and many others.

Are you ready to get started?

First off, be aware that this is not a portion-reduction plan. While your caloric intake will likely be reduced by replacing some of your old eating habits with new ones, it isn't the main goal, and you won't be left ready to gnaw your arm off in hunger. (Although if you're looking to deliberately cut calories, stay tuned for some weight-loss guidelines on page 94.) The *Beanalicious Living* plan includes replacing foods low in nutrients with, as Dr. Joel Fuhrman describes it, "nutrient-dense"

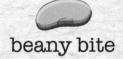

beany bite

Beans were considered an emblem of vitality by the ancient Egyptians, who strategically placed them in the tombs of the pharaohs for sustenance in the afterlife.

beany bite

*Many bean
types are rich in
folate, which
plays a significant
role in heart
health.*

alternatives. How fabulous is *that?* Real, healthy food is actually the most satisfying way to go!

Let's take a closer look at nutrient density. As I've discussed throughout this book, much of what we *think* we know about nutrition is actually based upon the "facts" that allow industry to sell more products. But as numerous studies prove, it's the whole-foods engine that's driving the health train, so we're going to review some of the key components. Food nutrients work in harmony—synergistically—which means that whole foods like an apple are actually *more* than the sum of their core, peel, and seeds.

Specific nutrients that the apple contains, once extracted and placed into a pill or supplement, just don't deliver the same benefits that they do in whole form. You need a certain amount of nutrients and fiber to keep your body healthy and feeling satisfied; you can't just rely on calorie counts. You can eat a day's worth of packaged foods and take a lot of supplements to try to get your allotment, but if your goal is to look and feel fantastic, you best bet is on whole foods.

As Dr. Fuhrman explains, we rely on food for both nutrients to keep us healthy and calories for the energy we need. The problem is when we're ingesting lots of calories but without the right nutrients; we're missing those vitamins, minerals, phytochemicals, and fiber that keep our bodies satisfied. So you can chow down on a bowl of "fortified" cereal only to crave another round not long afterward despite the ample amount of calories your breakfast contains. This often leads to more eating, and a blurred understanding of what healthy satisfaction feels like.

Conversely, when we feed our bodies whole foods, like lots of fresh produce and legumes, we'll feel satisfied on far fewer calories and can more easily maintain stable blood sugar, higher energy levels, and a healthy weight *without* complicated calorie-counting plans. Studies on long-term weight loss have shown that an average of three—only *three*—people out of 100 were able to maintain calorie-cutting weight-loss success for more than five years. Are you going to be one of those three? I know I am. Because it's not lack of control that's keeping those other 97 people overeating.

The trick is to find the most nutritionally loaded food per calorie, which is remarkably easy; the answer is in plants. Dr. Fuhrman has coined a nifty acronym to help make this easy to remember. Think GOMBBS: greens, onions, mushrooms, beans, berries and seeds, which he advocates as menu staples every day. In fact, Fuhrman recommends a daily diet of 90% unrefined plant foods, which includes beans and grains, but not meat and dairy. I know it sounds extreme and maybe even unpleasant, but—just for kicks—let's check out what a day of that might look like using some of the Beanalicious recipes you'll find in Part 2.

Breakfast
Some choices: Easy Fruit and Nut Granola, Apple Crisp Oatmeal, a Super Sprout Smoothie, a Healthy Breakfast Burrito. Enjoy with a glass of lemon water, add some mate (a traditional South American beverage), green tea, or coffee, and you're off to a great start.

Snack
Raw veggies dipped in House Blend Hummus; a handful of raw almonds or a soy chai latte.

Lunch
Some choices: Betty's Bean Burrito, Springtime Quinoa topped with greens, a White Bean Caesar Salad, a Simple Rice and Bean Bowl; fruit or nuts.

Snack
Whole-grain crackers with Basic Bean Dip; a piece of fruit and a cup of green tea (hot or iced).

Dinner
Some choices: Crunchy Cashew Fennel Slaw with Curried Sweet Potato and Lentil Soup, Smoky Jo's Pinto Bean Sauté with a White Bean Caesar salad, Polenta Fiesta Layer Cake with Asian-style Green Beans, or a simple Snappy Veggie Stir-fry served atop Basic Brown Rice.

This food is delicious, inexpensive, and easy to make. Honest! And, even better, it's okay to eat it in abundance. When you move away from the 75% prepackaged-style meal that the average American consumes, you benefit from the abundance of nutrients that whole foods have to offer while at the same time liberating your body from the rash of chemicals, toxins, and further unknowns so prevalent in our industrial food system.

At this point you may be thinking, "Okay, but I'd love a little meat with it, too." The *Beanalicious Living* plan is, as I've mentioned elsewhere, flexitarian. The recipes were designed with bean, grain, and veggie bases, but meat and fish (I recommend that they be hormone- and antibiotic-free) can be added throughout. I also suggest keeping portion sizes in mind, too; more on that shortly.

And when you do replace meat with beans and plant foods, it's never at the expense of protein. As discussed in Chapter 11, concern about protein deficiency is the single most common misperception when it comes to a plant-based diet. Most foods contain protein in varying amounts, including and especially beans. And while animal foods and soybeans are the only ones that contain complete proteins all in one source, the body stores the protein components and combines the proteins you need from a variety of sources to create the exact same complete protein chain.

Protein recommendations vary depending on whether you cite researchers such as Dr. Fuhrman and Dr. Campbell, or more conservative sources such as the USDA MyPlate guidelines. With the Beanalicious lifestyle, I take the middle-of-the-road approach, advising you to tailor your protein requirements individually based on your needs. I'm comfortable with the Institute of Medicine's adult daily recommendation of .8 grams of protein for every kilogram of body weight per day. That's 58 grams for a 160-pound adult. Does it sound a little confusing? Not to worry. Personally I think this kind of exact analysis is overkill anyway.

In the U.S., we're averaging 15% of calories from protein, so on the standard 2,000-calorie-per-day diet, that's about 75 grams of protein, when 50 grams is the moderate recommendation. So most of us are weighing in at around 30% more protein than we really need. And remember, too much animal protein has been linked to a variety of negative health effects, including heart disease and cancer. As I've mentioned before, if this sounds like the opposite of what you've been taught about meat and dairy, it helps to keep in mind where most of that information came from.

If you're including animal protein in your diet, I advise cutting back to no more than two 3-ounce portions per day *at most*. That's about the size of two decks of playing cards or one entire average-sized burger. I know this suggestion can be a challenging one, especially when children are in the mix. Meat can be cheap and easy—just boil a hot dog, pop it into a bun, add some ketchup, and *voilàsimo!* And with regard to the color of your meat, as in red or white, it makes no difference as far as your health is concerned: meat is meat.

The problem with the average meat-centric meal—aside from all the saturated fat, simple carbs, and sometimes preservatives—is that with so few phytochemicals and nutrients, and so little fiber, it won't leave you feeling satisfied for long. Experts observe that only 5% of our daily caloric intake comes from the fresh fruit, vegetables, beans, nuts, and seeds we should be relying on for good health, while 40% comes from animal products. A swap in those statistics would go a long way toward good health; many nutrition experts suggest keeping our daily consumption of animal products under 10%.

So maybe you could replace that hot dog with an organic corn tortilla, black beans, brown rice, avocado, and your favorite salsa. You'll be getting fiber, vitamins, nutrients, complex carbs, and protein galore—without any of the other stuff that does a body bad. My guess is you'll find the whole-foods option infinitely more delicious, cost-comparable, and, once you've got your plan down, just as easy.

Beans, nuts, seeds, grains, and dark leafy greens like spinach and kale all contain high levels of protein per serving. Per calorie, spinach contains twice as much protein as a cheeseburger. So if you're eating a healthy diet rich in veggies, beans, and grains, you're getting enough protein. If you're *still* not sure, add a couple of tablespoons of hemp seeds to your juice or smoothie, and you'll gain 10 grams of protein.

Move Over, Prozac!

Here's another potential benefit to keep in mind. Researchers at the University of Melbourne discovered that women were 30% less likely to suffer from depression and anxiety while eating a diet rich in produce, whole grains, and plant-based proteins. Did you know the National Institute of Mental Health lists depression, categorized as a "Major Depressive Disorder," as the leading cause of disability in the U.S. for people ages 15–44? That's scary stuff.

I can relate to this statistic first-hand, having suffered from mild anxiety-induced depression for most of my adult life. But since I've switched away from refined foods and more fully into plant-based eating, I've never felt healthier or more alive. How liberating, how wonderful, how empowering it feels to have that veil lift where I never would have expected it.

It was this amazing change in my personal well-being that first motivated me to share healthy eating tips and recipes through the blogosphere. But the more I talked to other moms, the more frequently I heard the frustrations associated with too little time and few approachable recipe and menu-planning ideas. That's just one of the many reasons I'm thrilled to be sharing my Beanalicious tips and strategies in this book.

Not Milk?

Another longstanding diet myth is the calcium conundrum. For years we've been taught the importance of dairy foods for strong bones, and to fight osteoporosis. That's where calcium comes from, right? Just like protein has almost become synonymous with meat, milk has been pinned as the go-to source for calcium.

Yet this perception has been carefully orchestrated by some pretty convincing industry campaigning. The folks at the American Dairy Association—the same ones who brought us the catchy "Got Milk?" ads—work hard to keep the connection going. To further confuse the concerned eater, we're faced with an abundance of nutritional so-called news telling us we need dairy products, designed to present the statistics just the way they'd like us to hear them. While it's clear that our bodies do require calcium, ingesting dairy products, according to the Harvard School of Public Health, might not be the best way to get it. Studies show that consuming extra calcium appears to have no effect on bone density in adolescent girls and women.

Here's another reason to think hard about high-fat foods. A 12-year study conducted by the National Cancer Institute indicates that women who consumed one or more servings of high-fat dairy products per day had a 64% greater risk of fatality compared with those who consumed half a serving or less.

Fat concerns aside, another problem that has recently come to light with all dairy products, organics included, is the company they keep. High levels of Bisephenol-A (BPA) and phthalates have been measured in dairy products across the board. Apparently the equipment used to milk the cows, traditionally pliable plastics, contains these chemicals—which numerous studies have linked with impaired thyroid function, among other problems, as we covered in Chapter 8.

While most plant-based experts call milk a must-not, the Beanalicious perspective is that at best it's optional. Sixty-five percent of the world's population simply doesn't do dairy—without a problem. Here in the U.S., up to 50% of us are actually lactose-intolerant, and many don't even know it.

Some good alternative sources of calcium include fortified plant milks (organic rice milk is a family favorite), bok choy, and—yes— beans. Still, if you've *got* to have that Monterey Jack on your black-bean quesadilla, I suggest you limit it to one to two servings per day. (Don't forget to check your serving sizes.) And if you do opt for dairy products, make sure they're rBGH-free—because they aren't, unless specifically labeled so. The artificial growth hormone rGBH has been linked to breast cancer and other health problems in a number of studies, so why risk it?

Fiber Up!

Carbs are a big source of discussion these days, thanks to the infamous low-carb diet made famous by Dr. Robert Atkins. Carbohydrates are the starchy and sugary parts of food that break down into glucose, the sugar your body needs for fuel. However, not all carbs are created equal.

Complex carbohydrates, the type contained in fruits, greens, beans, and grains, are naturally low in calories and high in fiber. They're also an important part of a healthy diet. The fiber contained in complex carbohydrates, in addition to all the health benefits it offers, gives us the feeling of fullness that keeps us from overeating. And researchers have linked high fiber consumption with a lower risk of both cardio-vascular disease and type 2 diabetes.

Then there are the other carbs—the simple or refined version contained in white bread, white rice, pasta, pastries, crackers, most juices, and breakfast cereals. These tricky carbs cause a surge in insulin that leads to a kind of roller-coaster effect on blood sugar: way up, then way down. Insulin surges can create a cycle of hunger and overeating in the short term, and long-term are associated with weight gain, type 2 diabetes, and other health problems.

To your body, a cup of white rice is essentially the same as a teaspoon of sugar: quick to convert to glucose, then leaves you feeling hungry all over again. The Beanalicious philosophy is firm on this point: for positive health outcomes, choose complex over refined every time.

Whole grains—as in whole wheat, brown rice, and many of the foods made with those ingredients—fall into the complex carbohydrate family, and have a more leveling effect on blood sugar and insulin than do the whites. Since most women consume only about half the 25–35 grams of fiber most experts recommend, you may want to think about making the switch. Look for bread that lists whole wheat, whole rye, or some other whole grain as the first ingredient. Or, even better, buy bread that's made with only 100% whole grains, like 100% whole-wheat bread.

Sweet Enough Already

It's one of the biggest dietary dilemmas: how can healthy eating and a sweet tooth go hand in hand? The first step is to know your

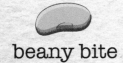

beany bite

Renaissance queen Catherine de' Medici is credited with introducing the white bean to France, which she brought along with Italian Chianti wine and olive oil during her journey to marry the future King Henry ll.

limits. The American Heart Association's recommended sugar intake for adult women is 5 teaspoons (20 grams) of sugar per day; for adult men, it's 9 teaspoons (36 grams) daily; and for children, it's 3 teaspoons (12 grams) a day.

Unfortunately, the average American eats about 22 teaspoons per day. Now I know you're not average, but the problem is, so does Big Food. That's why sugar is carefully disguised as HFCS (which we're on to, right?). As I mentioned earlier, sugar also comes under the guise of rice syrup, agave, cane juice, molasses, honey, and anything else they can get away with. But guess what? As far as your body is concerned, it's all just sugar. And as a result of the way it's hidden in so many processed foods, most people consume way too much.

Aside from the calorie factor, sugar taxes your immune system, accelerates the aging process, and—as discussed in Chapter 8—is highly addictive. Princeton University conducted some truly freaky studies demonstrating similar addictive properties in sugar and heroin, with both substances causing the same withdrawal symptoms in lab rats. That information alone is enough to scare me away.

What should you do if you're already hooked? First, don't panic! I've been there, too, so I can safely say that with simple step-by-step suggestions, you may find yourself cutting back without even realizing it. There are great-tasting plant-sourced substitutions such as stevia and sugar alcohol sweeteners. Not to be confused with the happy-hour version, these fermented sweeteners include xylitol, sorbitol, and erythritol. The resulting product is lower in calories than regular sugar and has actually been shown to help fight cavities, too.

I credit stevia as the only thing that worked to help me wean my way out of that scoop of sugar in my morning tea I thought I couldn't live without. Stevia does have a bit of an aftertaste, so once I kicked the sweetness habit, I went cold turkey and stopped using it, but it got me over the hump.

Instead of using white sugar or agave nectar for baked goods, I substitute local honey, molasses, or maple syrup whenever possible. While still recommended only in moderation, they do contain nutrients that will give you a little extra health boost. If you're feeling really adventurous, you might try experimenting with smart alternatives such as dates or applesauce for sweetening baked goods, since they still contain the fiber that keeps them from spiking your blood sugar and are easy to substitute for other sweeteners.

These alternatives are recommended to help bridge the gap while your taste buds resensitize as you eliminate refined foods from your diet. Eventually you won't believe you ever needed so much sugar to satiate your newly tamed sweet tooth.

Second, know where that extra sugar is hiding. Some of the biggest culprits are pre-made beverages such as sports drinks, juices, teas, and smoothies; check those labels diligently. More surprising are the foods you'd least expect to contain sugar—salad dressings, crackers, breads, and even pasta sauce often have hidden sweeteners. All processed and refined foods are potential culprits, so homemade, once again, is the surest route to low-sugar success.

Another thing that helped me was choosing whole fruits over processed juices—more fiber and less sugar. Luscious, sweet fruits such as cherries, grapes, and melon make a refreshing and wonderful dessert, and the natural fiber keeps that blood-sugar roller- coaster effect at bay. At our house we've switched from our morning cup of juice to water with a squeeze of fresh lemon and a dash of stevia for a healthy breakfast lemonade. My kids love it, and no one misses the sugar. Flavored tea is another great-tasting alternative to soda, and when it's caffeine-free it's kid-friendly, too.

Take it from a former sugar addict—this is a process worth under-taking. You'll look better, you'll feel better, and, soon enough, you may just forget those little white crystals ever existed.

Fats: All Bad?

Time for more nutrition myth-busting! This time we're going after "low-fat," because here again, not all fats are created equal. According to the Harvard School of Public Health, it's not the *percentage of calories* from fat, high or low, that's linked with disease, rather it's the *type* of fat you eat. The good fats, monounsaturated and polyunsaturated, are attributed with lowering disease risk. The bad fats, like saturated and especially trans fats, have been shown to increase disease risk.

Lots of processed food is manufactured to appeal to those of us who are interested in controlling our weight. As I've discussed, in this country obesity is big business, providing many new marketing opportunities for industrial food manufacturers (as well as for drug manufacturers). Simply adding the term "Low-fat" to a package can bring an instant increase in sales. But is it working? If you're a processed-food manufacturer, yes, it is, but it's becoming all too obvious that it's we consumers who sit squarely on the butt of that joke.

The FDA allows food manufactures to advertise the "Low-fat" label if their product contains 3 grams of fat or less per serving. This is the only piece of information that the low-fat label gives you. It doesn't say what's in the product, how it's made, or anything about the nutritional content, good or bad. We all know it's unhealthy to eat too much fat, so grabbing the low-fat alternative is the healthy option, right? That's what these crafty processed-food manufacturers are banking on. Sure, you cut back on fat per serving, but what about the rest?

The reality is that these foods are often supplemented with sugar, sodium, and other unhealthy additives to make up for the loss of flavor from the added fat. And what about those portion sizes? True to form, they're almost always reduced to fit the marketing goal. So your "3 grams of fat per serving" snack—which sounds so harmless—only adds up to 3.5 crunchy barbeque-flavor potato chips. Yeah, right, we'll only eat three before putting the bag back in the cabinet while we wait for our three more tomorrow!

The additives so prevalent in these low-fat foods are often the same ones that make it hard to stick to the portion size. No surprise, then, that the low-fat craze caused millions of us to actually *gain* weight by reaching for the "low-fat" but high-calorie carbs. Not a good trade-off.

You might be wondering, "What's the difference between good fats and bad fats?" It's a great question without a clear-cut answer. There are a wide range of opinions, even among the whole-foods, plant-based nutrition experts, about the health effects of fat. The big dispute seems to revolve around certain animal fats, which some whole-foods advocates argue are beneficial while others disagree. While all of the nutritionists referenced in *Beanalicious Living* agree that predominately plant-based diets are best, the animal protein/fat issue remains a, well, bone of contention. So let's look briefly at both sides of the argument.

Some fats are essential for maximum energy and optimum health, and whole plant foods contain many of them. Oils from plants such as olives and coconuts, nuts, seeds, and fish are especially high in good fats, although leading nutritionists disagree on whether these should be part of a healthy diet. Some of the experts I've consulted believe that plant oils and fats should be kept to a strict minimum and animal fats should be eliminated altogether.

Others believe that foods like grass-fed meat, eggs, and salmon, which contain specific forms of certain fatty acids, are essential for optimal health.

It's my philosophy that saturated fats, generally from animal-based sources, are best minimized or even avoided. Good fats such as plant-based mono- or polyunsaturated fats are healthy in moderation. In short, fat is still fat, and while some is healthier than others, handle with care.

Foods high in the Beanalicious "bad fat" category include processed meat, cheese, butter, and ice cream, along with processed foods made with trans fats derived from partially hydrogenated oil, which should *definitely* be avoided. Studies have shown a clear link between heart disease and the kind of trans fat found in Crisco, margarine, and many processed and fast foods. While the National Academy of Sciences has determined that no amount of trans fat in foods is safe, it can slip under the radar in low levels on food packages and is still used in fast-food restaurants.

While it's hard to steer clear of all saturated fats, all the time, the key once again is to say no to most refined, processed foods where you can. Remember, your saturated-fats mission, should you choose to accept it, is to keep those baddies to a minimum as best you can. Don't worry, you'll be so full of fiber it'll be a piece of cake . . . or at least a black bean brownie.

Got Salt?

Those who follow the Standard American Diet are no slackers on the salt intake: as a group, Americans are clocking in at double the recommended daily allowance of 2,500 milligrams per day. Almost 80% of this comes from the dire combination of refined/processed foods and eating out. "So what's wrong with a little extra salt?" you may be wondering. Well, for one thing, excess sodium has been linked in many studies to heart disease, high blood pressure, and stroke.

Worse yet, 70% of the U.S. population is considered at risk for, or predisposed to these salt-related diseases. If you're in this category, you should limit intake to 1,700 milligrams a day. But how to do it? Asking someone to count salt milligrams is just about as unrealistic as expecting her to keep a meticulous daily calorie tally—it's just not gonna happen.

In general the easiest way is to remove the real culprits from your diet altogether: say sayonara to junk food, and make a conscious effort to use less salt in your cooking. Keep in mind that you can lean into it. Err on the side of just slightly less salty, but add some salsa, lemon zest, or herbs to fill in the gap deliciously. Your tastebuds adjust the same way your eyes do to sunlight; today's low will soon be tomorrow's high. So hang in there!

The *Beanalicious Living* Top 10 Suggestions for Healthy, Unprocessed Eating

1. Most important: replace *refined and processed* with *fresh and whole* foods whenever possible.

2. Make lunch and dinner at least 50% raw or cooked veggies to start, and gradually up the percentage according to your comfort and satiation level.

3. Focus on fiber, as in whole-grain complex carbohydrates versus the refined white stuff.

4. Know your fats. Choose mostly unsaturated; limit saturated (as in

red meat and dairy); and avoid those trans fats! Plant oils, nuts, and fish are the healthiest saturated-fat sources.

5. Go plant-based over meat and dairy when you can. If you can't, stick to the 6-ounce-per-day portion which Harvard dietary guidelines recommend, and avoid factory farmed as much as possible.

6. Add beans to your diet in place of meat several times per week for ample protein and healthy fiber without the saturated fat.

7. Cut back on sugar and salt. Recommended daily sugar intake is 3 teaspoons for kids, 6 teaspoons for women, and 9 for men (down from the U.S. average of 22). One teaspoon of salt per day is a healthy guideline for adults. Avoiding processed foods and the table-salt shaker are two helpful ways to accomplish this goal.

8. Supplement with vitamin B12 and omega-3 fish oil or a daily dose of Neuromins DHA and a tablespoon or two of freshly ground flax seeds if you're avoiding animal products. B12 is the one nutrient plants don't provide, and according to leading nutritionists such as Dr. Dean Ornish, omega-3s are better assimilated by ingesting fish-oil products than plant-based alternatives.

9. Eat out less often. Restaurants, like any other business, need to maximize their profit margins, so lower-quality ingredients and lots of added fats are often the default.

10. Factor in lots of water, ample exercise, and plenty of self-appreciation for a job well done, every day!

Looking to Lose Weight?

As you may recall, the Beanalicious lifestyle isn't a weight-loss program per se, but the change from processed and takeout to whole-food, plant-based cooking often leads to easy weight loss. Since plants have so much more fiber than meat and dairy, a plant-based diet will fill you up faster, and with a greater range of nutrients and fewer calories. Tasty dishes like Mexican Caponata, Curried Chickpeas and Potatoes, Lentil Stuffed Peppers, and Mung Bean Crunch—you'll find these recipes, and lots more, in Part 2—are not only amazingly flavorful, these hearty bean-based dishes create a feeling of fullness which keeps you from overeating.

Sounds too good to be true, I know, but when you replace calorie-dense processed foods with nutrition-packed, high-fiber whole foods, you simply can't eat as much—no calorie- counting required. An independent scientific review compiling data from 87 different sources attributes a vegetarian diet to long-term weight loss in study participants. Vegetarians have a significantly lower rate of obesity and the related diseases that go along with it. Studies found that with all other factors held equal, vegetarians weigh an average of 3–10% less than meat-eaters.

Remember, this is not an all-or-nothing approach. If you're uncomfortable cutting out all animal products, try reducing your meat consumption and you'll still experience positive changes. Personally, I refrain from eating meat, but I do enjoy a bit of locally churned goat cheese or some sustainably caught seafood now and then. The heart of the Beanalicious approach is to avoid nutritionally devoid or high-calorie, low-fiber foods. How can you tell? Yep, they usually come in a package.

People often ask me what I eat to maintain a high level of energy and a lean, mean body weight. Because I'm not the type of gal to prioritize skinny over sustained energy, or expedience over flavor, I've put a lot of effort into creating a health (and weight) maintenance plan that places satisfaction as top priority, with ease of use as a close second.

Of course, replacing the processed with healthy whole foods is the crux of this plan, but I'm happy to share some simple no-starve tricks for kicking extra calories to the curb for good.

Beanalicious Living Top 10 Tips for Hunger-free Weight Loss and Management

1. **Rethink your drinks**. Americans on average consume an extra 350 calories a day from packaged drinks. Switching to water (plain or, if you like, fruit-infused) and unsweetened tea or coffee will help those

pounds to melt away. Even artificially sweetened "diet" beverages are linked with obesity and other health problems. Don't risk it! Naturally harvested stevia is a great option when you need a little something sweet.

2. **Harness your willpower**. As new research shows, willpower is like a muscle that tires, but can also be strengthened. By recognizing what your goals are—such as better health, more energy, and/or weight loss—you set the stage for making change. The more you make positive choices, the more likely you will be to make them in the future; so even when you slip up, get back on the bus and keep on going!

3. **Always shop with a plan**. Decide what your weekly menu will look like and create your grocery list based on that. The *Beanalicious Living* sample grocery list is available both in this book and online—feel free to use it. (You can find it at http://www.Elizabeth-Borelli.com.) Don't buy anything that doesn't belong in your body, no matter how good a deal it is this week. And never shop on an empty stomach.

4. **Eat breakfast**. Studies show that people who eat breakfast daily ingest fewer calories overall than those who hold out until lunchtime. The National Weight Control Registry reports that "successful losers"—people who have maintained a 30-pound (or more) weight loss for at least a year—make breakfast a daily habit. Whether it's a Super Sprout Smoothie, Brown Rice Breakfast Pilaf, or homemade granola that you crave, pencil in breakfast for a healthy start.

5. **Exercise**. Physical activity is as effective as Zoloft in reducing depression and its benefits extend far beyond that. Circling back to the willpower effect, research reveals that regular exercise not only helps us feel better, it builds willpower, too. Whether it's a brisk walk around the block, a bike ride to the store, or a yoga class on your lunch break, fit it in every day if you can.

6. **Eat mindfully**. This isn't some zany New Age idea. A small but growing number of studies show that taking the time to stop, sit down, and focus on what you're eating helps prevent both overindulgence and unhealthy choices. Try enjoying the first five minutes of your meal in silence (and appreciation!), take small bites, and chew thoroughly

to help slow things down; eating more slowly gives your body the 20 minutes it needs to process satiety so that you're tuned into fullness signals before it's too late.

7. **Skip the "diet" foods**. As touched on earlier in this book, companies are legally permitted to list health and weight-loss claims on packaged foods with little regulation, lots of room for exaggeration, and often out of context. Most often these products are stripped of natural fiber and nutritive properties, which are later added back in with a host of other unwanted ingredients, so your vitamin-fortified blueberry cereal bar contains some of the nutrients of whole blueberries, but artificial colors, high-fructose corn syrup, and preservatives, too. No processed food is healthier than the caloric equivalent of the whole food it's made from, and no magic product will make you lose weight.

8. **Replace the oils in your diet with less calorie-dense alternatives**. Applesauce or mashed bananas make delicious substitutes in baked goods, there are endless options for oil-free salad dressing, and cooking without oils is a snap. The options are endless, and delicious enough that you won't miss a thing, especially those excess calories. See the *Beanalicious Living* recipe section in Part 2 for options galore.

9. **Wipe out the whites**. Refined white (or processed wheat) bread, rice, pasta, and, of course, most sweet treats are stripped of their natural fiber during processing, which leaves them so rapidly digestible that your body immediately converts them to sugar. Instead, opt for whole-grain foods which require the body to break down fiber before converting starches to sugar, allowing slower, healthier assimilation for lasting energy without the carb crash.

10. **Keep your meals full of variety and your plate half-full of fiber**. Calorie-dense and/or fatty foods such as high-fat meat and dairy should be treated as condiments, with bean, whole-grain, and veggie-based dishes taking center stage as the main event. With the *Beanalicious Living*'s sensible, scrumptious menu suggestions, it's easy to maximize your enjoyment of good, healthy food without extra calories.

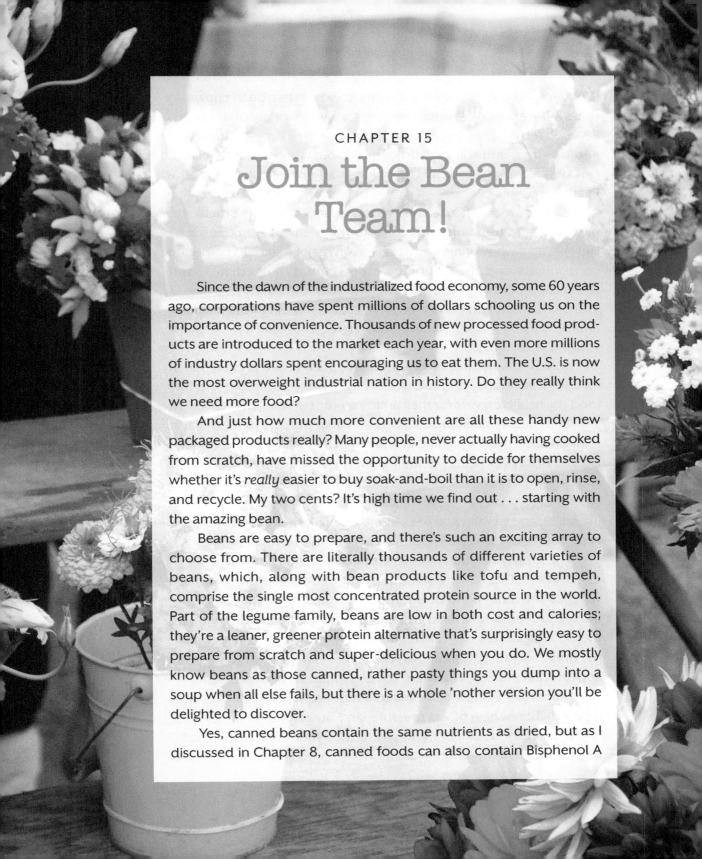

CHAPTER 15

Join the Bean Team!

Since the dawn of the industrialized food economy, some 60 years ago, corporations have spent millions of dollars schooling us on the importance of convenience. Thousands of new processed food products are introduced to the market each year, with even more millions of industry dollars spent encouraging us to eat them. The U.S. is now the most overweight industrial nation in history. Do they really think we need more food?

And just how much more convenient are all these handy new packaged products really? Many people, never actually having cooked from scratch, have missed the opportunity to decide for themselves whether it's *really* easier to buy soak-and-boil than it is to open, rinse, and recycle. My two cents? It's high time we find out . . . starting with the amazing bean.

Beans are easy to prepare, and there's such an exciting array to choose from. There are literally thousands of different varieties of beans, which, along with bean products like tofu and tempeh, comprise the single most concentrated protein source in the world. Part of the legume family, beans are low in both cost and calories; they're a leaner, greener protein alternative that's surprisingly easy to prepare from scratch and super-delicious when you do. We mostly know beans as those canned, rather pasty things you dump into a soup when all else fails, but there is a whole 'nother version you'll be delighted to discover.

Yes, canned beans contain the same nutrients as dried, but as I discussed in Chapter 8, canned foods can also contain Bisphenol A

(BPA), a synthetic estrogen, exposure to which has been shown to disrupt the endocrine system and trigger a wide variety of disorders. BPA concerns aside, bulk beans are less expensive; sodium- and additive-free; and will get you comfortable with how truly easy it can be to cook from scratch, which is an important part of the Beanalicious journey.

When you learn how easy it is to take back some of the methods, practices, and traditions we've lost to the media-driven consumer lifestyle, it's empowering. You'll realize you're not a slave to corporate concoctions and their dubious claims, empty ingredients, and chemical processing. You can become your own Betty Crocker—a more stylish, health- savvy version, that is—freeing your culinary creativity using the simple, everyday ingredients that work best for you and your family.

Both beans and lentils pack a healthy, plant-based protein punch for a lot less (money *and* calories). They're often called the "perfect food" by health experts for their amazing nutrient profile. An excellent source of dietary fiber, protein, and iron, many beans are also rich in folate, which plays a significant role in heart health. Beans contain dozens of key nutrients, including a few that most of us could use more of—potassium, calcium, and magnesium. And depending on the type of bean you choose, you'll also get decent amounts of vitamins B1 and B2, and vitamin K as well. Kidney, pinto, and mung beans are a great source of those all-important omega-3 fatty acids.

These tasty health dynamos also deliver a megadose of antioxidants. The USDA's ranking of foods by antioxidant capacity lists three varieties of beans—pinto beans, red beans, and red kidney beans—at the top four among all food groups. Not only are beans nutrient-rich, they're a natural calming and regulatory remedy as well. They contain the amino acid tryptophan, which studies have shown to regulate appetite, aid in sleep, and even reduce symptoms of depression.

Numerous studies tie beans to a reduced risk of heart disease, type 2 diabetes, high blood pressure, and breast and colon cancers. "Certain key foods can dramatically reduce your heart disease risk," says Dr. Dariush Mozaffarian, an associate professor at the Harvard

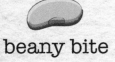

beany bite

School of Public Health. In one study, people who ate legumes such as beans and lentils at least four times a week had a 22% lower risk of heart disease than people who ate them less than once a week.

Aside from the nutritional benefits, beans are the perfect "go to" basic because you can find them practically everywhere; plus, they're easy to store, simple to prepare, and very versatile. This humble staple really *is* as close to a perfect food as you can find. From spreads to soups to salads, to just served plain with olive oil and salt—which is the way my kids eat them—you'll never run out of new recipe ideas.

One concern some people have about beans is . . . the music they've been known to generate.

No worries! I've got some easy tips to keep those beans gas-free. Soak your beans overnight and rinse well before cooking. Aside from lentils, most varieties cook for about an hour. And really, it's hard to overcook most legumes, so just keep them boiling until they're soft (which often takes longer than you think). Tossing in a few cumin or fennel seeds, a bay leaf, a slice of fresh ginger, or a three-inch strip of dried kombu seaweed during cooking can also make a huge difference.

If you're still plagued by "digestive issues," try the Quick Soak Method described on page 155, which breaks down those sugary starches with maximum efficiency so you can enjoy your beans without the aftermath.

And finally, keep in mind that it can take some time for your body to acclimate to a diet based more on plant proteins than meat proteins. A few months of persistence can pay off with a stronger, calmer digestive tract and trouble-free bean-eating.

Ready to begin the *Beanalicious Living* adventure? Grab some reusable bags, prep your big glass storage jars, jot down your shopping list, and you're on your way back to home-style living, your way.

Getting Started

Bill Phillips, fitness expert and author of *Body for Life*, says, "When we fail to plan, we plan to fail." As I've mentioned elsewhere, planning ahead makes it all doable. With everything that's going on in my life, the last thing I have patience for is sitting down and trying to plan a complicated weekly menu requiring a long list of specific ingredients. I like having options and choices, but without a framework to keep it manageable, I know I'd end up right back where I started, and no closer to achieving my goals.

Just like anything you build from scratch, the key to a healthy meal is a solid foundation. Keep in mind this basic maxim: the more processed the food, the less nutritious. Beyond that, cooking from scratch knocks an easy 30% of average caloric intake right off the top when compared to a restaurant or takeout, and is less likely to contain ingredients you wouldn't use in your own kitchen either. Bottom line: keep it simple and cook at home.

And even if the closest Chinese takeout phone number tops your speed-dial list, don't panic. Change can take time and it's sometimes easier to implement in stages. Start by reaching just outside of your comfort zone and see how that goes. Before you know it, you've reached a new goal and you're ready to grow again—especially once the health benefits begin to pay off.

What works for me is to allocate a little preparation time on the weekend for my weekday meals; it's infinitely easier to pull it all together over the next six days, even if some last-minute prep work is still required. For example, every weekend I cook a pot of quinoa and another of black beans that I use as a base for my lunches throughout the following week. It's fast, healthy, delicious, and cheap. And I apply this same principle to dinners just as easily.

This is the beautiful thing about bean dishes made from scratch. When they're not going solo, they work well in so many dishes that you always have flexibility in meal preparation. You can use the ingredients you have on hand, or venture out and get more creative as time, opportunity, and appetite dictate. I determine my bean and grain recipes weekly. Based on what I come up with, I soak the beans on Saturday (for those that need soaking), cook them on Sunday, and that becomes the basis for meals galore during the week.

At the heart of the Beanalicious lifestyle is the reality that beans are easy—really easy!—to prepare from scratch. If you can boil water, you can cook beans. No secret skills or stealthy ingredients required. Then, for less than the cost of a six-pack of diet Coke, you've got the basis for a delicious, protein-rich meal.

I typically go with favorites like kidney or black beans, garbanzos, navy beans, or lentils, since these are both diverse and readily available. Prepare enough beans for three or four dishes, so if you cook black beans, plan to use them for, say, a Healthy Breakfast Burrito, tossed into a Corn and Black Bean Salad, folded into a Wrap and Roll, or tucked into a Jewel and Bean Bake.

Another advantage to beans is that they have a long shelf life, even after cooking. I like to boil up a batch to use over the next three or four days as my culinary spirit moves me. I'll often use them in a lovely bean and green sauté on the first evening, then refrigerate the rest to toss them in salads over the next few days, as well as to include in a wrap or tortilla for a lunch or two.

Otherwise, pop any leftovers into the freezer, where they'll last nicely for up to three months, then simply put them in the fridge to thaw the night before or on the counter the morning before you're ready to use them. It's easy once you know what to do. So take a chance, grab a pan, and learn to love your beans!

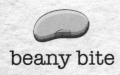

beany bite

Consider the sprout: sprouts are super-nutritious, containing up to 100 times more enzymes than most raw foods, enabling your body to extract more vitamins, minerals, amino acids, and essential fats per calorie.

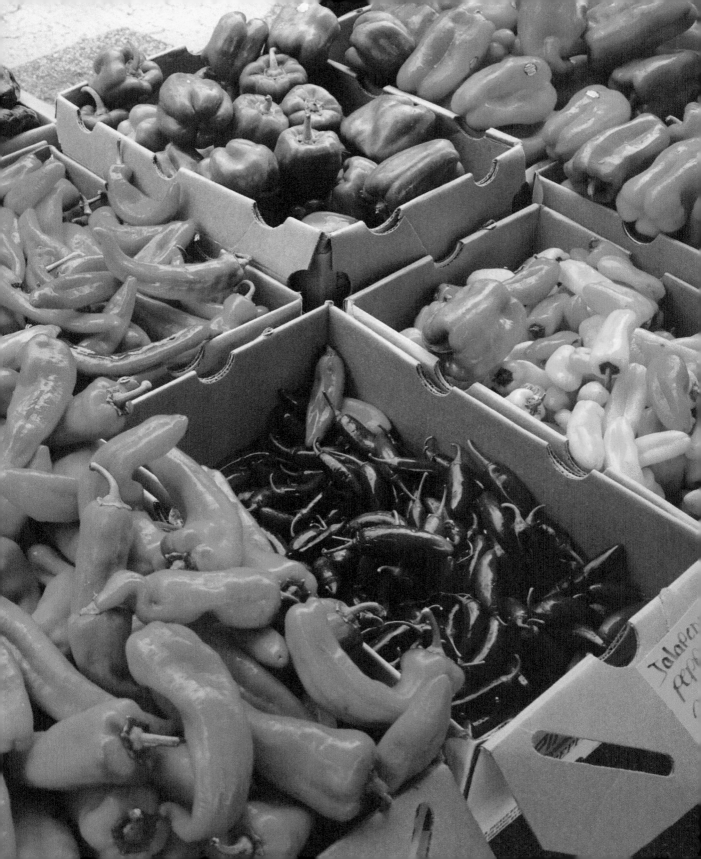

PART 2

The Beanalicious Solution:

Preparation Guide & Recipes

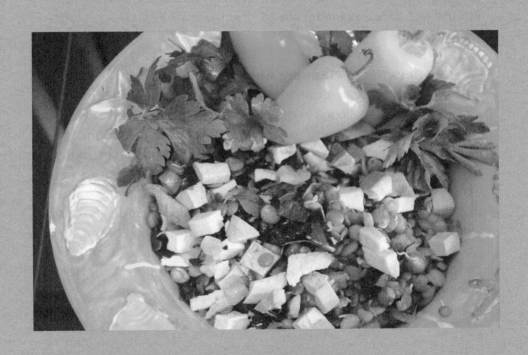

CHAPTER 16

Get to Know Your Beans

In the beginning, planning a meal can seem intimidating, but it's actually really easy to plan your meals around the perfect culinary trio comprised of a bean, a green, and a grain. Dress these up with a few good accessories: a sauce, dressing, or spice blend, then top it off with a portion of protein and you're on your way to a culinary masterpiece (or at the very least, a really good nosh). The *Beanalicious Living* recipes were created for ease of use: short lists of readily available ingredients, simple preparation methods, and everyday cooking tools are the key. But the real trick is planning ahead, and there are Beanalicious tools for that, too.

The Benefits of Planning Ahead

You'll see the bean recipes grouped by variety on page 121, making it simple to soak and cook in quantity to use for more than one dish during the week. So if you're going to make Black Bean Soup, for example, you might want to plan on making a Jewel and Bean Bake or maybe some Caribbean Black Beans that week, too. Some bean varieties, like mung and adzuki, don't require soaking, so if you skipped that step you don't have to go beanless! Just choose accordingly today while you get tomorrow's soak on. Want a handy Bean Soaking and Cooking Chart for easy reference? There's one on page 116, and you can also stop by my website at http://www.ElizabethBorelli.com for a downloadable version.

A Label of Love

In any situation where you're looking to make changes that stick, it's really helpful to remove the obstacles to success. In the case of home cooking, it's the extra preparation steps that can threaten to stop you in your tracks and turn you back to old habits.

At first glance, it might seem that the extra soaking and cooking steps required in bean preparation are the big obstacles, but pouring beans and water into a pot and turning on the stove are too easy to be relegated to that category! So maybe it's the extra legwork: looking up soak times or finding the right page in a cookbook to get the prep info you need. It can be a hassle! But luckily, you can avoid lots of extra steps and streamline it all.

How? With some simple planning ... *and* some self-adhesive labels, available at your local office-supply store or even your mainstream grocery store.

These handy labels will help you get all the information you need in the most visible location: on your food containers. I always keep labels on hand in my cooking space and you may want to also; if you buy anything in bulk, ever, you're gonna need them. And if you're in a DIY mood, visit http://www.ElizabethBorelli.com and go to the "Label It" link. Grab a sheet of blank labels and print out some stylish Beanalicious labels for your bulk beans, designed to display soaking and cooking instructions right there in plain sight. Before you know it, cooking beans from scratch will be a breeze.

Getting Organized

Chapter 19 contains preparation instructions, a sample menu, and shopping lists, all designed to simplify the process. If it sounds easy, it is! Once you get to know your beans, weekly meal planning will work to make life easier, instead of the other way around.

Bean Varieties

There are more than two dozen varieties of bean common to the United States. Selected for easy use and wide availability, the Beanalicious recipes incorporate nine of these, which I'll describe below—but this list is just to get you started. Other scrumptious possibilities like lima beans, gigantes, and black-eyed peas are no less alluring, and it's easy to find recipes galore for those, too. And, if you're lucky enough to have access to local heirloom bean varieties, I highly recommend you give them a try. Unique to your region, these native varieties can be substituted for many of the Beanalicious recipes; just factor in changes in cooking times.

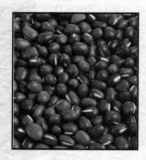

Adzuki beans

These small red-brown beans have a nutty, sweet taste. Popular in Japanese cooking, they're lower in fat and higher in protein than most varieties. They're delicious in rice dishes, or when sprouted and used in salads or stir-fries, often in place of mung beans. Soak overnight, simmer on the stovetop for 40 minutes, or skip the soaking step and simmer on the stovetop for 1¼ hours until tender.

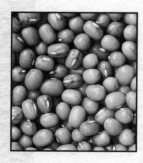

Mung beans

These delicate little beans range in color from yellow to black, but you'll find the green variety most commonly in the bulk section of your local health-food store. Frequently used in Asian cooking, the mild mung bean is often eaten sprouted as well. Soaking is optional. To cook, simmer on the stovetop for 40 minutes, or if you opted to skip the soaking step, simmer on the stovetop for 1¼ hours until tender.

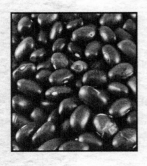

Black beans

A widely popular bean, black beans are often used in Latin American and Southwestern-style cooking. Also known as turtle beans, these creamy-textured legumes are quite versatile due to their mild flavor (think black-bean brownies), and are wonderful added to rice dishes and salads for an extra protein punch. Soak overnight and simmer on the stovetop for 1½–2 hours until tender.

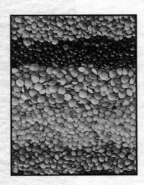

Lentils

A rich, nutty legume with roots in the Middle East, this group includes several varieties to choose from. Green or brown lentils and the smaller red lentils are the types most commonly found in your local bulk bins. You don't need to soak these, unless you're sprouting, and they cook more quickly than other bean varieties, too. Simmer green or brown lentils for 25–35 minutes on the stovetop. Black, or French, lentils are slightly firmer and more flavorful than the green/brown variety; they'll cook in 20–30 minutes.

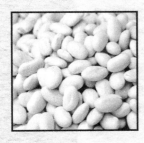

Navy (or white) beans

Sometimes known as white beans, these small beans are versatile enough to use in chili, soups, and stews, often in place of cannellini beans, which taste very similar. Instead of kidney beans, try these for a delicious New England–style baked bean alternative. Soak overnight, simmer 1½–2 hours, rinse, and drain.

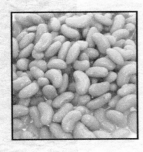

Cannellini beans

Often used in Italian cuisine, these white kidney beans retain their shape after cooking, so they're perfect for adding a mild nutty flavor and palatable texture to soups, salads, and pastas. Soak overnight, then bring to a boil on the stovetop for 10 minutes before reducing the heat and simmering for 1½–2 hours.

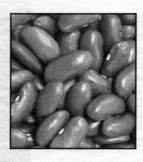

Kidney beans

These creamy red beans are delicious paired with rice, enjoyed in a chili, or cooked up Boston baked–style. They're also quite interchangeable with black beans, so substitute freely in equal quantities. Soak overnight and simmer on the stove for 1½ –2 hours.

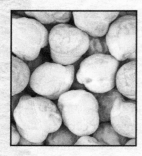

Garbanzo beans

Also known as chickpeas, these nutty, full-bodied beans are much more delicious when soaked and cooked than out of a can. A vegetarian staple in the UK and India, garbanzo beans are an excellent source of zinc, folate, and protein. Soak overnight, rinse and drain, then cook for 2–3 hours on the stovetop. You almost can't overcook them.

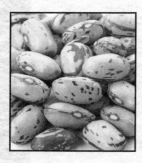

Pinto beans

Mellow, sweet, and creamy, pinto beans are named for their mottled, brownish-red topcoat. A close cousin to the kidney bean, they can be substituted in most recipes by simply adding an extra 15 minutes to cooking. To prepare, soak overnight and simmer on the stove for 1½–2 hours until tender.

CHAPTER 17

Adventures in Sprouting

Every time I teach a sprouting class I hear the same thing from the older participants in the crowd: "I was a master sprouter back in the day; can't believe I stopped doing it!" Sprouting is indeed a bit of a lost art, and I'm delighted to include a chapter on this recently reemerging and extremely valuable culinary practice.

Sprouts are just your everyday seeds, beans, or grains taken to the next level in terms of nutrition and deliciousness just by soaking, rinsing, and allowing them a few days to germinate—that is, sprout—before eating. While you can find many sprout varieties at most health-food stores, growing them yourself is fun, easy, and much less expensive. You'll also avoid the contamination problems which can occur with commercially grown varieties.

Sprouted foods are not only nutrient-rich, they're easier for your body to digest and absorb as well. Sprouts contain significantly higher quantities of enzymes than even raw produce, which enable your body to extract more of the nutrients you need from the food you eat. Both the quality of the protein and the fiber content improve during sprouting, too. And these superfoods can be grown in your kitchen for less than the price of a latte— just add water!

I originally discovered the wonders of seed and bean sprouts at my local farmers' market. With their lively taste appeal *and* tremendous health benefits, it wasn't long before I was hooked. One sprouting class and dozens of recipes later, I developed my own Green Sprout Kit and accessories to help make kitchen sprouting easy and convenient. (See the Resource section on page 213 for more information.)

I prefer jar sprouting over the other commonly used methods such as sprouting trays and bags. Jars let you go plastic-free, keep the cleanup easy, and don't require much counter space—all of which makes the process manageable. Which is great for busy people with small kitchens, like me!

Want some tips on growing your own seed and bean sprouts? Read on! If you're not quite ready to give it a try, you can buy them pre-sprouted at your local farmers' market, health-food store, or main-stream grocery store.

Your home-grown sprouts are up-to-the-minute fresh and delicious. All you need to grow them right in your kitchen is some seeds, jars, and screens. That's it!

Getting Started

Beginner Varieties

Any seed, bean, or grain is sproutable, but some take a bit more know-how. Easy seed choices are alfalfa, mustard, radish, and clover. Or you might start with legumes. Lentils, mung beans, garbanzos, and green peas are all good choices. Even wheat, in the form of wheat berries, is easy to sprout, and adds a whole new level of nutrients to baked goods.

Sprouting Selection

Choose your seeds base on taste preference. If you like the small, green sprouts such as alfalfa, which are often used in salads, sand-wiches, and spring rolls, start with seeds. If you prefer legumes (beans, lentils, peas), which are great in a stir-fry, salad, or soup, start there. Sprouted legumes taste much the same as the dried varieties, but require much less cooking time than dried. They are also more tender and easier to digest. I suggest giving them a try if you haven't already— you may be pleasantly surprised!

The legumes you use should be "seed quality," rather than "food quality." Seed-quality legumes are cultivated for sprouting, while food quality are meant for cooking in their dry, unsprouted state, and tend to have a lower germination rate.

Fortunately it's becoming easier to find seeds, beans, and grains specifically grown for sprouting. These can be found in most health-food stores, often right in the bulk bins or specialty shops, and are also available online. Once you have your seeds in hand, store them in airtight containers until you're ready to use them; glass jars work well for this purpose.

Setting Up

Growing supplies

Wide-mouthed 1.5-quart Mason jar with 2-part lid
Stainless steel screen or fiberglass mesh to cover
  the mouth of the jar
Sprouting bag or towel to cover your sprouting jar
Dish rack or flat shallow containers for the jars to drain into
Finding space

During the germination process, sprouts, like most seeds, prefer a dark, temperate (60–85 degrees) location, away from drafts and direct heat. You can sprout right on your kitchen counter by just covering your jar with a sprouting bag or towel to keep the light out.

Step-by-Step Sprouting

1. Measure out your seeds or beans. In general, 1 ounce of seeds yields about 1 cup of spouts, so ¼ cup (for a 2-cup yield), seems to be a good starting point for small seed sprouts since they have a short shelf life. Soaked beans and legumes expand to approximately double the volume as when dried, so plan accordingly.

2. Place seeds in a mesh strainer or in your sprouting jar and rinse with tap water, then drain.

If you used a strainer for rinsing, pour seeds or legumes into your Mason jar. Fill the jar three-quarters full with water, cap with mesh screen and lid, and let soak overnight (if prepared in the evening) or for the following times:

small seeds:	5–14 hours
larger seeds or legumes:	8–18 hours
grains:	10–16 hours

For more seed-specific soak, rinse, and germination details, take a look at the Sprout Chart on page 130.

3. After soaking, drain the water and rinse the seeds thoroughly. The soaking water is said to contain natural toxins released from the seeds during germination, so rinsing two to three times a day is recommended.

4. After each rinse, place the jar upside down and tilted at a 45-degree angle in the spot you've selected and cover with a sprouting bag or towel. The goal is to keep the seeds/beans damp—and not soaking in water—until they sprout. You can maximize their sprouting times by keeping them in a suitably warm, dark location.

5. Let the spouts germinate for the suggested number of days (see chart on page 113). Sprout most seeds 1 to 2 inches; grains up to 4 inches; and beans ¼ to 1 inch. You may want to vary growth time depending on your plans for their use. Shorter sprouts are great for eating whole, but you'll want them longer if you plan to use them for juice.

6. With small seeds, once they've sprouted, you can place the jar in strong, indirect sunlight for two to three days to allow them to develop some nutrient-rich chlorophyll (Skip this step for legumes, though).

7. When the jar is full and the sprouts or legumes are ready to use, store them in an airtight container—a capped sprouting jar is fine—in the refrigerator. Be sure your sprouts have drained for at least five hours before storing, as too much moisture can cause spoilage.

Sprouting experts recommend that small seeds be hulled, with their shells removed, before placing them in the refrigerator. It's easy to do by soaking in a large bowl of water where hulls will float to the top for easy removal.

Beginner's Sprout Chart

For use with the jar method

Seed or Legume	Quantity	Soaking time	Rinses	Ready in
Alfalfa seeds	⅛ cup	6–14 hours	2–3 per day	4–6 days
Adzuki beans	1 cup	8–12 hours	2 per day	3–5 days
Garbanzo beans	2 cups	12–18 hours	2–3 per day	2–4 days
Lentils	1 cup	8–12 hours	2–3 per day	2–4 days
Mung beans	1 cup	8–18 hours	2 per day	3–5 days
Whole green peas	1½ cups	8–15 hours	2 per day	3–5 days
Radish seeds	⅛ cup	6–10 hours	2 per day	3–5 days
Broccoli seeds	⅛ cup	6–10 hours	2–3 per day	4–6 days
Soft wheat berries	2 cups	8–14 hours	2–3 per day	3 days

Once you get the hang of it, sprouting can be rather addictive. You'll find new ways to enjoy sprouts just so you have an excuse to keep them growing! And when you're feeling even more adventurous, check out the more advanced, detailed sprouting chart at http://www.ElizabethBorelli.com.

CHAPTER 18

Preparation Made Easy

The Beanalicious mantra is that beans are simple to prepare. Wait till you see just how true this is! Beans are so easy, in fact, that whether you're using dried or pre-cooked, it's hard to go wrong (and harder still to overcook them).

Easy Guidelines for Successful Bean Cooking

1. Begin by rinsing beans in cold water. Most beans require soaking for up to eight hours or overnight for thorough cooking and increased digestibility. Soak your beans in enough tap water, at room temperature, to cover by at least 3 inches of water. Beans expand to up to two and a half times the size of dried, so plan accordingly. After soaking overnight, if you don't cook them that day, replace the soaking water, refrigerate, and cook the next day.

2. Drain soaking water and replace with fresh, room-temperature tap water for cooking. Beans should be covered by at least 3 inches of water during cooking.

3. Increase digestibility with de-gassing herbs. A couple tablespoons of dried bay leaf or the Mexican cooking spice epazote are very effective, or add a piece of kombu (a type of seaweed) during cooking to pre-neutralize any potential digestive problems.

4. Bring beans to a simmer and cook uncovered for the recommended time based upon variety, or until tender. Stir occasionally and add more water if needed.

5. Wait until beans are fully cooked to add salt, but you can add 1 tablespoon of olive oil to the beans during cooking to reduce foaming and prevent boiling over.

6. Remove beans from heat and let cool in the cooking water to keep them from drying out.

Beans last up to five days in the refrigerator once cooked, but freeze well for up to three months and thaw quickly, especially when added to hot soups or stews.

Store dried beans in an airtight container—jars are perfect for this purpose—in a cool, dry environment, away from direct sunlight, for up to 12 months.

The Quick Soak Method

If you're in a hurry, here's a super-quick preparation suggestion. It's also the most effective de-gassing method I know.

In a large saucepan, cover dried beans with three times their volume of water and bring to a boil. Boil for 2 minutes. Remove from heat, cover, and let stand for 1 hour. Drain.

Refill the same saucepan with an equivalent measure of water to beans. Again bring beans to a boil, reduce heat, and simmer, covered (adding extra water if necessary), for about 45 minutes to 1¼ hours, depending on the type of bean you're using. Drain and enjoy in your favorite, bean-friendly fashion.

Spice up Your Beans

Certain seasonings will make your beans sing, rely on them and you'll rarely go wrong. Some of my favorite spices for beans are garlic, parsley, cumin, thyme, basil, oregano, fennel, and pepper of any kind, but truth be told, it's hard to go wrong no matter how you spice it. I typically use 1 teaspoon of seasoning per 2 cups of cooked beans. Mix, match, and taste away—you'll soon develop your own favorite combinations. I also add salt to beans after cooking: ½ teaspoon salt per 2 cups of cooked beans, but this is optional, of course, and variable to taste.

You may choose to add 1 tablespoon of oil. Olive, walnut, or coconut oil are good options, depending on the flavor profile you choose. Perhaps finish this off with some tomato sauce or salsa; ⅓ cup per 2 cups cooked beans is a nice ratio. Top your beans with chopped cilantro or shredded cheese for easy homemade goodness.

Bean Soaking and Cooking Chart

Bean Variety	Dry : Cooked	Soak Time	Simmer Time
Adzuki Beans	1 : 3	Optional	40–50 minutes (if soaked), or 1¼ hours
Black Beans	1 : 3	8 hours or overnight	1½–2 hours
Black Eyed Peas	1 : 3	Optional	20–30 minutes (if soaked), or 45–55 minutes
Cannellini Beans	2 : 3	8 hours or overnight	1½ hours
Garbanzo Beans	1 : 4	8 hours or overnight	1½– 2½ hours
Kidney Beans	1 : 2	8 hours or overnight	1½ hours
Green Lentils	1 : 2	Optional	25–35 minutes (if soaked), or 45 minutes
Red Lentils	1 : 2½	Not recommended	15–20 minutes
Black Lentils	1 : 2	Not recommended	20–30 minutes
Mung Beans	1 : 3	Optional	45 minutes (if soaked), or 1–1¼ hours
Navy or White Beans	1 : 3	8 hours or overnight	1½– 2 hours

- Drain water after soaking and use fresh water for cooking beans.
- Beans are best cooked in a large, covered pot.
- Use 3–4 cups of water for each cup of dried beans. The water should be 3–4 inches above the top of the beans.
- Don't add salt or seasoning to the cooking water; this can be added after beans are cooked.
- Keep beans cooking at a low simmer until done.
- Do not undercook—give your beans the time they need to fully soften.
- Read about the Quick Soak Method (page   ) for the best way to reduce hard-to-digest complex sugars.

CHAPTER 19

Simple Steps to Beanalicious Menu Planning

This chapter will help you to get from reading the recipes and thinking how nice it would be to enjoy them, to actually having a plan, acquiring the ingredients, and making it happen. Lovely as it will eventually be to have all your wholesome meals dialed in with time to spare, it's a learning process, so patience and gentle persistence are equally key. Remember, there are 21 meals in a week, so it helps to determine your initial goal from there. Stay within your comfort zone to start, but just barely. You'll build new cooking habits just like any other habit, and when you stick with it, this challenging course will become a walk in the park before you know it.

As I've mentioned before, the key is to prepare in advance. Ready? Let's walk through the steps.

Ten Simple Steps to a Week of Beanalicious Meals

1. Read through the *Beanalicious Living* recipes on pages 128–208 for inspiration. You can also start by choosing some dishes listed in the Bean Varieties chart on page 121. Channel your adventurous side and include some things you haven't tried before!

2. Select three to five bean dishes you want to try, using two or three bean varieties. For example, I'll soak a pot of garbanzo beans and one of white beans to use for House Blend Hummus, North African

Date Tangine, a chopped veggie salad with Lemon Cumin Dressing, Mediterranean Kale and Bean Sauté, and Minestrone Soup. Two beans, five dishes. Whether you choose your recipes based upon the beans you have on hand, or select your beans based on the recipes that you can't wait to try is up to you—just have fun!

3. Using your selections from Step 2, plug your three to five dishes into your weekly menu. Create your own or download one at http://www.ElizabethBorelli.com, then duplicate and improvise wherever possible. For example, this evening's Snappy Veggie Stir-fry with Ginger Peanut Sauce will make a quick and yummy lunch tomorrow packed atop some leftover brown rice or quinoa. You'll be able to fill in as many as 10 spaces this way.

4. Add a grain dish you can commit to preparing from scratch, either from the Beanalicious recipes, your personal repertoire, or from any other source that inspires you.

5. Select two sauces to prepare ahead to use during the week. The Beanalicious sauce recipes are perfect for pulling together a last-minute stir-fry, creating a quick pasta topping, or dressing a hearty salad. Of course, as with the grain dishes, feel free to use any other sauce recipes that you like.

6. Add three to five recipes to your weekly menu plan, based on your selections in Step 5, to your menu below. Duplicate freely to fill up to 10 spaces.

7. You should have between 6 and 15 recipes entered into your weekly menu plan. Fill in the rest with whatever sounds good to you, keeping it whole foods–based as much as possible. Once your weekly menu plan is complete, or at least as close as you're going to get it, use it with your Beanalicious Shopping Guide (available at **http://www.ElizabethBorelli.com**) to create a list and get your shop-

ping done in preparation for the week ahead. Three tips I swear by: never shop on an empty stomach; always ignore store promotions which can lead to impulse buying; and stick to your list!

8. Set aside some time on Friday evening or Saturday to soak your beans overnight. If you're sprouting, this is a good time to start soaking your beans or seeds for that purpose as well.

9. Schedule additional time over the weekend to cook your beans, wash or chop veggies, and prepare sauces. An hour is plenty; you can do your prep work while your beans cook.

10. Store beans, veggies, and sauces in the fridge and freezer. You're ready for a week of delicious home cooking!

Sample Beans, Grains, and Sauces List

2–3 beans:	garbanzo beans
	white beans
	black beans
2–3 grains:	quinoa
	kamut
	brown rice
2 dressings/sauces:	Lemon Cumin Dressing
	Cilantro Mint Sauce

Beanalicious
Living

Sample Menu Using Selected Beans, Grains and Sauces

Recipes in italics indicate a Beanalicious recipe

	Monday	Tuesday	Wednesday	Thursday	Friday	Saturday	Sunday
Breakfast							
	Super Sprout Smoothie	*Brown Rice Breakfast Pilaf*	*Super Sprout Smoothie*	*Healthy Breakfast Burrito*	*Super Sprout Smoothie*	*Apple Crisp Oatmeal*	Tofu scramble
	Easy Fruit and Nut Granola	Fruit	*Easy Fruit and Nut Granola*		Fruit	Fruit	
Lunch							
	Lemony Broccoli	*Mexican Caponata*	*Thai Cabbage Salad*	*Savory Ginger Carrot Soup*	Spinach salad	*Springtime Quinoa*	Green salad
	Polenta Fiesta Layer Cake	*Curried Brown Rice*	Quinoa	*Springtime Quinoa*	*Fennel, White Bean, and Collard Green Sauté*	*Orange, Fennel, and Kamut Salad*	Minestrone Soup
Dinner							
	Nutty Brussels Sprout Curry Sauté	*Thai Cabbage Salad*	Green salad	Spinach salad	Green salad	*White Bean Caesar Salad*	
	Curried Brown Rice	*Parsnip Adzuki Fried Rice*	*Savory Ginger Carrot Soup*	*Fennel, White Bean, and Collard Green Sauté*	*Simple Bean and Green Soup*	*Polenta Fiesta Layer Cake*	Out with friends!
	Mexican Caponata	*Snappy Veggie Stir-fry, Cilantro Mint Sauce*	*Springtime Quinoa*	Steamed kamut	*Orange, Fennel, and Kamut Salad*	*Lemony Broccoli*	

Review the menu options from the list below or by reading through the recipe section on pages 128-208. Choose your bean and grain varieties and your recipes.

Bean Variety	Recipe Suggestions
Adzuki beans	Parsnip Adzuki Fried Rice
	Zesty Five-bean Salad
Black beans	Mexican Caponata
	Caribbean Black Beans
	Healthy Breakfast Burrito
	Easy Beanie Chili
	Black Bean Soup
	Jewel and Bean Bake
	Polenta Fiesta Layer Cake
	Vegetarian Fajitas
	Basic Three-bean Salad
	Betty's Bean Burrito
	Corn and Black Bean Salad
Cannellini beans	Beany Bruchetta
	Sweet Potato and White Bean Chili
	Simple Bean and Green Soup
	Pasta with Cannellini Beans and Arugula
	Minestrone Soup
	Savory Ginger Carrot Soup
Garbanzo beans or Chickpeas	House Blend Hummus
	Beanalicious Garbanzo Bean Salad
	Curried Chickpeas and Potatoes
	North African Date Tangine
	Sicilian Garbanzo Marinara
	Mediterranean Kale and Bean Sauté
	Basic Three-bean Salad

Mung beans	Harvest Salad
	Zesty Five-bean Salad
	Quinoa Garsnippity
Navy or White beans	Beany Bruchetta
	Mediterranean Kale and Bean Sauté
	Fennel, White Bean, and Collard Green Sauté
	White Bean Caesar Salad
	Sweet Potato and White Bean Chili
	Simple Bean and Green Soup
	Minestrone Soup
	Savory Ginger Carrot Soup
Kidney beans	Easy Beanie Chili
	Vegetarian Fajitas
	Basic Three-bean Salad
	Savory Baked Beans
	Betty's Bean Burrito
	Meatless Refried Beans
Pinto beans	Easy Beanie Chili
	Meatless Refried Beans
	Smokey Jo's Pinto Bean Sauté
Green lentils	Lentil Stuffed Peppers
	Agape Salad
	Curried Sweet Potato and Lentil Soup
Red lentils	Red Lentil Kitcharee
Sprouts	Sprouted Wheat Breakfast Cookies
	Kale, Sweet Potato, and Sprout Salad with Miso Dressing

Mung Bean Crunch
Super Sprout Smoothie
Fresh Thai Spring Rolls with Ginger
   Peanut Sauce
Agape Salad
Spicy Sprout Salad
Red Lentil Kitcharee

Grain Variety	Recipe Suggestion
Brown rice	Basic Brown Rice
	Lemon Cumin Rice Salad
	Curried Brown Rice
	Veggie Fried Rice
	Brown Rice Breakfast Pilaf
	Snappy Veggie Stir-fry
	Simple Rice and Bean Bowls
	Wrap and Roll!
Quinoa	Springtime Quinoa
	Quinoa Tabouli
	Snappy Veggie Stir-fry
	Simple Rice and Bean Bowls
	Wrap and Roll!
Barley	Barley Pilaf
	Snappy Veggie Stir-fry
	Simple Rice and Bean Bowls
	Wrap and Roll!
Kamut	Orange, Fennel, and Kamut Salad
	Snappy Veggie Stir-fry
	Simple Rice and Bean Bowls
	Wrap and Roll!

Basic Kitchen Tips and Tools

One of the secrets to successful home cooking is a well-stocked pantry. It's reassuring to know you've got the resources on hand to whip up a meal right then and there. Another secret of success? It involves the tools of the trade. You can't create a masterpiece without access to at least the basic materials. So I've created some lists of a few simple standbys to keep right at your fingertips—for the pantry, the spice rack, and the kitchen workspace.

Pantry

I'm rather particular about my cooking liquids, because that's where a lot of chemicals and unhealthy fats lie. Included with this short list of healthy and flavorful cooking oils, condiments, and vinegars is one simple instruction: use sparingly.

Tamari
Bragg Liquid Aminos
Rice vinegar
Coconut oil
Olive oil
High-heat grapeseed oil
Walnut oil
Sesame oil (keep refrigerated)
Nondairy cheese (I like the Daiya brand)
Aged balsamic vinegar
Asian fish sauce (for non-vegans)
Stevia
Honey
Molasses
Maple syrup

Spices

This is my go-to list, and you'll probably have some favorites of your own, so adjust as needed. Store your spices in airtight containers away from direct sunlight. Spices never go bad, but they do lose their flavor after a while, so give anything over a year old the sniff test. If it's out of scent, it's time to replace it.

Dried bay leaf, epazote, or kombu (add to simmering beans
  to increase digestibility)
Whole peppercorns in a grinder
Powdered or granulated garlic (I buy this in bulk from
  my local market; it's fresher)
Fresh garlic
Ground ginger root
Fresh ginger root
Ground cinnamon
Ground cumin
Dried thyme
Ground coriander
Whole coriander seeds
Italian seasoning blend
Ground curry
Dried dill
Ground turmeric
Chipotle powder
Wasabi powder
Nutritional yeast

Other Condiments

These can be lifesavers when you're down to carrots and onions, fresh out of sauces, and in need of a meal in 20 minutes or less. Add a jar of salsa to a batch of beans and *voilà*— instant delish! Roasted red peppers and cashews make a quick and tasty sauce, and some sunflower seeds can bring the most basic of salads up a notch.

Jarred organic salsa
Jarred or BPA-free canned tomato sauce
   (I like the Muir Glen brand)
Roasted red peppers
Jarred capers
Spicy brown mustard
Organic ketchup (most non-organic brands contain
   high-fructose corn syrup)
Horseradish
Red curry paste
Bouillon (I like the Better Than Bouillon brand)
Whole-grain pasta
Tahini

Cooking Tools

As I may have mentioned, I'm a minimalist. I've enjoyed cooking during my entire life, yet my culinary tool collection remains pretty basic. I don't own a juicer or a fancy food processor, not even a Crock-Pot. While never one to dispute the glories of a great kitchen gadget, I find that a good-quality blender (or Vitamix, if you can swing it), a few sharp chefs' knives, and a small array of decent-quality pans will get you through most recipes without a hitch. Basics aside, my tool list is relatively short—with just enough to get the job done. However, if gadgets are what it takes to get you going, by all means, acquire accordingly!

Large hand grater, stainless steel, freestanding
Small hand grater, stainless steel (for fine grating)
Cutting boards, one large and one small
    (I recommend bamboo)
Stainless steel colanders, one large and one small
Spice grinder or mini food processor
Good-quality vegetable peeler
Stainless steel garlic press
Glass or stainless steel hand-held juicer
Stainless steel kitchen shears
Stainless steel potato masher
2-cup glass measuring cup
Set of stainless steel measuring spoons
Kitchen timer
    (or any timer you can comfortably use in the kitchen)
Self-adhesive labels (visit http://www.ElizabethBorelli.com
    for a free downloadable template)
Apron (your kitchen tool belt)

What about Organic?

I'm often asked, "Does everything need to be organic? What about foods like lemons, which have peels to protect them from pesticides?"

I believe that organic is preferable. However, in terms of both price and availability, it's not always an option. My quick rule of thumb: sweet and thin-skinned produce is better to buy organic, as are spinach, potatoes, and lettuce; they tend to absorb more pesticides which are difficult to completely wash away. Thick-skinned produce like citrus fruits, bananas, and avocados, as well as broccoli, cauliflower, and onions, are fine to buy conventionally grown if organic isn't possible.

For more information, visit the website of the Environmental Working Group, a very helpful consumer advocacy group, at http://www.ewg.org.

CHAPTER 20

Beanalicious Recipes

In this chapter I'm excited to share some of my favorite recipes. You can follow the cooking and seasoning directions as noted, but do feel free to get creative by varying the ingredients as the urge strikes you. You simply can't go wrong!

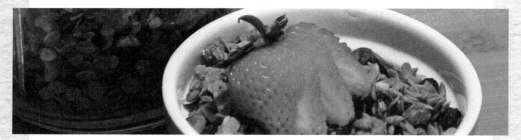

Breakfast

Aptly named the most important meal of the day, studies show that breakfast-eaters weigh less and focus more than those who skip it. And high-quality whole foods are the healthiest way to start your morning. Here are some easy recipe ideas to rise and shine with.

Super Sprout Smoothie
3 to 4 servings

Join the green juice revolution! Leading nutritionist and author David Wolfe calls this his best piece of dietary advice, and he keeps his simple with cucumber, parsley, celery, and lemon juice. Martha Stewart calls green juice her secret to gorgeous skin, and uses spinach, ginger, and orange peel as standard ingredients. "Wellness warrior" Kris Carr offered my first introduction to the stuff, and provides many versions of her go-to health beverage in her fun and fabulous book *Crazy Sexy Diet*. With so many options and so much positive health evidence, I highly recommend you give this super bev a try.

The Beanalicious version suggests adding your choice of nutrient-dense, high-protein sprouts to bring a spring to your step and a glow to your fabulous face every time—no caffeine required. Ingredient choices are flexible, but be sure to keep it fresh, raw, and mostly green to avoid sugar overload. The chia seeds and Spirulina add the super-charge; don't skip them.

Although it's best to drink this smoothie right away, it also freezes well.

Ingredients:
- 2 organic celery stalks, leaves optional
- 1 organic green apple, cored
- 1 cup fresh alfalfa sprouts
- 2 cups or ½ head curly kale, stems removed
- ½ cup fresh parsley
- ½ cup fresh or frozen organic raspberries or pineapple
- 2 tablespoons chia seeds
- 2 tablespoons Spirulina powder
- 4 cups water
- 1 teaspoon stevia

Rinse the produce and toss it with the other ingredients in a blender or Vitamix; blend until smooth.

Healthy Breakfast Burrito
1 serving

A favorite especially among kids and surfers, this hearty combo offers a healthy way to enjoy your leftover beans for breakfast. Simple, satisfying, and—of course!—delicious, this burrito is loaded with all the protein you need to get your day off to a great start. Multiply the ingredients by the number of people you're feeding, keeping in mind that the recipe below serves one generously.

Ingredients:
- 1 whole-grain tortilla
- ¼ cup cooked black beans, precooked, and still warm or reheated
- 3 tablespoons salsa (organic if possible; jarred is an easy alternative)
- ¼ cup tofu (optional)
- 3 tablespoons guacamole or mashed avocado
- Chili powder and salt to taste

To cook beans: soak for at least 8 hours or overnight. Drain and rinse beans, then add to a large stockpot; fill with water to 6 inches over the top of the bean blend. Turn heat to medium-high and bring to a low boil, then reduce heat to simmer and cook for 1½ to 2 hours. Drain and rinse.

Mash tofu with some chili powder and salt in a small bowl. If beans need to be heated, add them to a small saucepan with 2 tablespoons of water and heat for 3 to 5 minutes until warmed through.

Warm your tortilla using one of these easy methods:
- Place the tortilla in a dry (oil-free) stainless steel skillet over medium heat and cook for about 30 seconds each side.
- If you're doing more than one, try the oven method. Wrap a stack of 2 to 5 tortillas in aluminum foil and place in a preheated 350° oven until heated through, 15 to 20 minutes.

Layer the warm tortilla with the bean mixture, salsa, and guacamole or mashed avocado, then spread evenly in a line down the center. Fold in the ends and roll.

Brown Rice Breakfast Pilaf
1 serving

I discovered this delicious concept during a weekend retreat at the world-famous Esalen Institute in Big Sur, California. They serve brown rice for breakfast daily with dishes of nuts, raisins, and coconut flakes available on the side to include (or not). It's so simple, healthy, and yummy that it's become a favorite we enjoy regularly at home.

Ingredients:
- 1 cup brown rice (short- or medium-grain)
- 1 to 2 teaspoons cinnamon powder
- 1 teaspoon salt
- ½ cup each or in any combination: chopped walnuts or pecans, raisins or dried cranberries, coconut flakes
- 2 tablespoons honey, maple syrup, or stevia (optional)

Prepare rice by bringing 2¼ cups of water to a low boil in a large saucepan. Add rice and return to a boil before reducing heat to low and covering the pan. Simmer for 45 minutes or until all water is absorbed. Remove from heat, add remaining ingredients, and serve.

Easy Fruit and Nut Granola
10 servings

As it turns out, granola is one of those things so easy to make, that once you learn you'll wonder why anyone would ever feel the need to buy it. Once you get the basic recipe down, you can experiment with spices, nuts, and dried fruit to find your favorite flavor combination. Enjoy it served with a scoop of stevia-sweetened yogurt (plant-based or dairy) for a light, easy, and super-healthy breakfast, or pack some to go for a midday or lunchbox snack.

Ingredients:
- 3 cups steel-cut oats (or any blend of rye, barley, or spelt flakes can be substituted)
- 2 cups raw mixed nuts: pecans, walnuts, almonds, cashews, or pumpkin seeds are good choices
- 1 teaspoon salt
- 2 teaspoons cinnamon
- ½ teaspoon ground ginger
- ½ cup walnut oil

- ½ cup honey or maple syrup
- 1 teaspoon vanilla
- ¾ cup raisins or dried cranberries

Preheat oven to 350°. In a large mixing bowl, combine oats, nuts, salt, and spices. Stir to combine. Add in oil and honey or maple syrup and vanilla, and mix thoroughly. Pour the mixture onto a baking sheet (rimmed if you have it) and bake for 30 to 40 minutes, stirring every 15 minutes or so to ensure even cooking. Remove from the oven and stir in dried fruit. Let cool for at least 15 minutes before serving.

Store in an airtight container for up to 1 week.

Apple Crisp Oatmeal
4 servings

I make this for my kids as a special treat. (Yes, cooking on a school morning is my version of a special treat!) Chop the apple the night before and toss in some lemon juice to keep it from browning; it'll save you precious prep time in the morning.

Ingredients:
- 2 cups steel-cut oats, or any combination of spelt, triticale, rye, or barley flakes
- 1 tablespoon coconut oil
- 3 cups boiling water
- 1 apple, cored and diced
- 1 to 2 teaspoons cinnamon
- 1 teaspoon salt
- 3 tablespoons honey or maple syrup, or 1 teaspoon stevia
- ¼ cup organic soy or almond milk creamer
- ½ cup walnuts

In a large sauté pan, heat coconut oil and add apple. Sauté on medium heat for 1 minute, then add oats and sauté for 2 to 3 minutes longer. Add boiling water and reduce heat to medium-low (or simmer).

Cook for 30 minutes or until water is absorbed. Turn off heat and let stand for 5 minutes longer. Add remaining ingredients and serve.

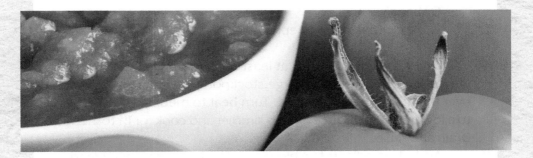

Light Bites

These simple, nutritious, whole-foods recipes are perfect for a light lunch (for you or the kids) or as appetizers or anytime snacks.

House Blend Hummus

Makes 2 cups

There's no big secret to making good hummus. If you puree garbanzo beans in a blender, it tastes good. Add some seasonings and it tastes great. Here's a favorite basic recipe, but feel free to experiment by adding other ingredients (roasted red pepper, black olives, or cooked butternut are my top picks) and/or seasonings of all sorts. As I've said before: as with most bean dishes, you can't go wrong.

Lots of hummus recipes call for tahini, but I like this lighter version as a nice alternative. It's a great dip for veggies, and I also love this as a wrap or sandwich spread. Delish!

Ingredients:
- 2 cups garbanzo beans, precooked
- 2 tablespoons lemon juice (fresh if available)
- 2 tablespoons walnut or olive oil
- ½ to ¾ teaspoon salt

- 2 cloves garlic, minced; *or* 1 teaspoon powdered or granulated garlic

Optional:
- ½ cup roasted red peppers

To cook beans: soak for at least 8 hours or overnight. Drain and rinse beans, then add to a large stockpot; fill with water to 6 inches over the top of the bean blend. Turn heat to medium-high and bring to a low boil, then reduce heat to simmer and cook for 1½ to 2½ hours. Drain and rinse.

Add all ingredients to a blender or food processor and blend until smooth. Add water if needed for blending, but final consistency should be very thick. Store refrigerated up to 5 days.

Basic Salsa
Makes 2 cups

Salsa is a bean's best friend! I use it to flavor many of my bean dishes, especially where rice is involved, or as a favorite dip for chips. This simple recipe makes fresh salsa almost as easy as opening a jar.

Ingredients:
- 2 large tomatoes, diced
- 1 cup onion, diced
- 1 cup water
- 1 clove garlic, crushed; *or* 1 teaspoon powdered or granulated garlic
- 1 teaspoon salt
- 1 teaspoon lime juice (fresh if available)
- 2 tablespoons cilantro, chopped (a blender or mini food processor makes the prep work easy)
- 1 teaspoon chipotle powder (optional)

Place onion in a small bowl. Boil 1 cup water and pour over onion. Let stand for 1 minute, then drain and mix in remaining ingredients. Let stand for at least 15 minutes before serving.

Southwest Style Salsa
Makes 2½ cups

This simple salsa combines black beans, avocado, and corn for a scrumptious accompaniment to tortilla chips. It's also a delicious addition to a green salad or a tasty topping for your favorite grains.

Ingredients:
- 1 ripe avocado, peeled and diced
- 1 cup black beans, precooked
- ½ cup fresh or frozen organic corn
- 1 teaspoon lime juice (fresh if available)
- ½ teaspoon salt
- ½ teaspoon powdered or granulated garlic
- ½ teaspoon chipotle powder

To cook beans: soak for at least 8 hours or overnight. Drain and rinse beans, then add to a large stockpot; fill with water to 6 inches over the top of the bean blend. Turn heat to medium-high and bring to a low boil, then reduce heat to simmer and cook for 1½ to 2 hours. Drain and rinse.

Combine all ingredients in a mixing bowl and serve.

Red Pepper Cashew Spread
Makes 2 cups

This creamy spread is a flavorful addition to any sandwich or wrap. You can also serve it atop crusty whole-grain bread or crackers for a tasty snack or starter. Try it in a pita pocket stuffed with last night's leftover salad for a light and easy lunch.

Ingredients:
- ½ cup Cashew Cream (see page 146); *or* ¾ cup raw cashews, soaked for at least 30 minutes (or up to 8 hours) in enough water just to cover them, then drained
- 1½ cups roasted red peppers (jarred is fine; be sure to drain)
- 1 teaspoon salt

- 2 cloves garlic; *or* 1 teaspoon powdered or granulated garlic
- 1 tablespoon Bragg Liquid Aminos
- 1 tablespoon rice vinegar

Place all ingredients in blender or food processor and puree until smooth. Store refrigerated for up to 1 week.

Basic Bean Dip
Makes 2 cups

This dip is wonderfully simple to prepare, and better yet, you can make it using any bean variety. It's delicious served as a dip for veggies, a topping for Beany Bruschetta (see recipe below), or as a sandwich spread. Double or triple the recipe and keep leftovers in the fridge for up to 1 week.

Ingredients:
- 1½ cups beans (white, garbanzo, and black beans are favorites, precooked)
- 2 tablespoons olive oil
- 2 tablespoons water
- 2 cloves garlic; *or* 1 teaspoon powdered or granulated garlic
- 1 teaspoon salt
- 1 teaspoon dried sage or thyme (optional)

Add ingredients to a blender or food processor and puree until smooth.

Note: See the Bean Soaking and Cooking Chart on page 116 for bean preparation instructions.

Beany Bruschetta

A quick and tasty appetizer, perfect for parties. It's especially good made with navy or cannellini beans.

Ingredients:
- 1 whole-grain baguette
- 2 to 3 tablespoons olive oil
- ½ cup bean dip
- ½ cup tomato, diced

Preheat oven to 350°. Slice the baguette lengthwise. Brush the entire surface lightly with olive oil and place, cut side up, in the oven. Bake for 5 to 10 minutes until lightly toasted. Remove from heat and spread with a thin layer of bean dip. Top with chopped tomato, and serve immediately.

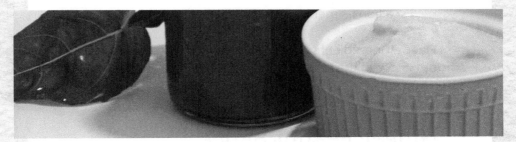

Spices, Sauces, and Dressings

Spice blends, sauces, and dressings are a mainstay in Beanalicious cooking; when combined with veggies, beans, and/or grains, they make it simple to create a delicious meal in very short order.

These are easy to prepare in larger quantities, and I recommend having at least two always on hand. Choose your favorites to create stir-fries, rice and bean dishes, or super-quick lunch wraps. They're also great with pasta or over salads. Dip your veggies in 'em, or spread atop fresh, whole-grain bread. You'll find dozens of uses and, I'm sure, more than one family favorite!

Cilantro Mint Sauce
Makes 1½ cups

This fresh herb blend is a super addition to any rice or grain dish. Inspired by Indian cilantro chutney, it will add terrific flavor to all things vegetable, so use it as an excuse to get creative in the kitchen. With fresh, whole ingredients you can't go wrong.

Ingredients:
- 1 serrano chili pepper, seeds removed (optional)
- 2 bunches cilantro leaves
- 1 cup mint leaves
- 4 tablespoons lime juice (fresh if available)
- 1 tablespoon Bragg Liquid Aminos
- 1 teaspoon salt
- 1 teaspoon sugar
- 6 scallions, greens removed

Place all ingredients in blender or food processor and blend until smooth. Store in the refrigerator for up to 1 week, or in the freezer for up to 3 months.

Ginger Peanut Sauce
Makes 2 cups

This sauce will make your plain brown rice noodles sing. Toss in some chopped scallions, broccoli florets, and mung beans for a lovely Asian-inspired dish. Or stir-fry your favorite veggies, toss in some of this scrumptious sauce, add some brown rice, include a side of Bean Sprout Salad (see page 155), and you're in for a truly great meal.

Ingredients:
- 2 inches ginger (unpeeled is fine, and feel free to guestimate your quantity)
- 1 clove garlic; *or* ½ teaspoon powdered or granulated garlic

- 1 tablespoon maple syrup
- ⅓ cup peanut butter
- 2 tablespoons white miso
- 2 tablespoons sesame oil
- 1 tablespoon rice vinegar
- 1 tablespoon Bragg Liquid Aminos
- ¼ cup water
- 1 teaspoon chili pepper powder or red pepper flakes

Place all ingredients into a blender or food processor and blend until smooth.

Vegan Curry Sauce
Makes 4 cups

This is a simplified version of the luscious curry sauces used in Indian cooking, but delicious still and perfect to prepare ahead and freeze for use when you need it. Some of the oil can be replaced with coconut milk, although it can be hard to source a non-canned (or BPA-free canned) version. Keep in mind that while the coconut oil adds flavor, it's also high in saturated fat, so find the calorie/fat balance that works for you. I like to add some heat with cayenne pepper or chili powder, but be sure to go easy—a little goes a long way!

Ingredients:
- 2 large onions, peeled and coarsely chopped
- 6 cloves garlic, peeled
- ¼ cup coconut oil
- 3 cups water
- 2 teaspoons curry powder
- 2 teaspoons ground ginger or 1-inch piece of ginger root (unpeeled is fine)
- ½ cup raw cashews, soaked in just enough water to cover them, for at least 30 minutes

Optional for added heat:
- 1 teaspoon chili pepper or cayenne powder
- 2 tablespoons red curry paste (available in the Asian section of most grocery stores)

Add 1 inch of water to a saucepan. Add onions and garlic and cover, turn heat to medium, and cook for 5 to 8 minutes, until onions are softened and translucent. Let stand for 5 minutes longer, then pour the hot mixture into a blender or food processor and add the remaining ingredients. Puree until smooth. This sauce freezes for up to 2 months, or can be stored in the refrigerator for up to 1 week.

Easy Mole Sauce
Makes 3½ cups

This is a tasty take on traditional mole, the richly spiced Mexican dish made extra-delectable with a touch of unsweetened cocoa. My version is much simplified, and made using vegetable bouillon in place of traditional chicken stock. Pour over your favorite stir-fry and serve up with brown rice for a delightfully different dish.

Ingredients:
- 1 onion, peeled and halved
- ½ cup pumpkin seeds
- 3 cloves garlic, peeled
- ¼ cup raisins
- 2 teaspoons vegetable bouillon
- 1 cup water
- ½ teaspoon cinnamon
- 1 teaspoon ground coriander
- 1 teaspoon ground cumin
- 1½ cups tomato sauce or puree
- 2 tablespoons unsweetened cocoa powder

In a medium saucepan over medium heat, cover and steam onion, raisins, and pumpkin seeds in water-bouillon blend for 5 minutes, until onion is soft. Remove from heat; stir in spices. When the mixture has cooled down enough to manage, pour into a blender or food processor and puree until smooth. Pour back into the saucepan, add tomato sauce and chocolate, and heat to a simmer. Cook for 5 minutes longer and serve.

Savory Sauce Blend
Makes 1¼ cups

This is a staple in my kitchen since it's so easy and versatile, plus the flavor blend is superb. More of a base than a finished sauce, I typically season it further with garlic, ginger, or sesame oil (or all three), but since the Savory Sauce Blend has such a long shelf life, I save steps by blending this ahead and adding finishing touches at cooking time. (I find it's a big help to label and date the bottle or container I store it in.)

Ingredients:
- ½ cup Bragg Liquid Aminos
- ½ cup rice vinegar
- 4 tablespoons Asian fish sauce

Blend all 3 ingredients and store in an airtight glass container for up to 6 months.

Lemon Cumin Dressing
Makes ½ cup

This highly flavorful dressing contains more oil than I generally use, but a little goes a long way, so use accordingly. The zesty flavor combination is lovely over greens and is also delicious when combined with rice or grains. Simple to make, it stays fresh in the refrigerator for up to 2 weeks.

Ingredients:
- ¼ cup lemon juice (fresh if available)
- 2 teaspoons ground cumin
- 2 teaspoons salt or Asian fish sauce
- ⅓ cup walnut oil
- 1 teaspoon powdered or granulated garlic

Combine all ingredients until fully blended. Store in a glass jar (labeled and dated) for future use.

Green Goddess Dressing
Makes 1¼ cups

This classic blend is lovely over a fresh garden salad, and makes a delicious dip for fresh veggies, too.

Ingredients:
- ⅔ cup raw cashews, soaked in 1 cup of water for at least 30 minutes before using
- 3 tablespoons fresh parsley (equivalent to a small handful)
- ¼ cup scallions, coarsely chopped
- ½ teaspoon salt
- 3 cloves garlic, peeled; *or* 1½ teaspoons powdered or granulated garlic
- 2 tablespoons Savory Sauce Blend (see page 141); *or* 1 tablespoon Bragg Liquid Aminos, 1 tablespoon rice vinegar, and 1 teaspoon Asian fish sauce
- 2 tablespoons lemon juice, fresh if available (optional)

Pour cashews and soaking liquid into a blender or food processor. Add remaining ingredients and puree until smooth. Store in a glass bottle in the refrigerator for up to 1 week.

Ginger Miso Dressing
Makes ½ cup

This is the dressing flavorful enough to transform iceberg lettuce and cello tomatoes (remember those?) into delicious cuisine in certain Japanese restaurants. Imagine how good it'll be with fresh organic greens or mung bean sprouts.

Ingredients:
- ¼ cup white or yellow miso
- ¼ cup tahini
- 2 tablespoons water
- 2 teaspoons powdered ginger; *or* ½ to 1 teaspoon fresh ginger, finely grated
- 2 tablespoons sesame oil
- 2 tablespoons rice vinegar
- 1 tablespoon Bragg Liquid Aminos or soy sauce
- Juice of ½ orange (approximately ¼ cup)
- ½ to 1 teaspoon salt (to taste)

Combine all ingredients and serve. Stays fresh in the refrigerator for up to 10 days.

Tahini Vinaigrette
Makes 1½ cups

This savory dressing does wonders for any vegetable salad, and is also wonderful drizzled over rice and served with a side of garlicky greens. Add some tofu or bean salad for a simple, wholesome meal.

Ingredients:
- ¼ cup water
- 3 tablespoons raw tahini
- ¼ cup olive oil
- ¼ cup lemon juice (fresh if available)
- 2 teaspoons tamari or Bragg Liquid Aminos

- 1 clove garlic; *or* 1 teaspoon powdered or granulated garlic
- 2 tablespoons maple syrup
- ¼ cup onion, coarsely chopped
- 1 teaspoon salt

Blend all ingredients in a blender or food processor until smooth, then serve. Store (labeled and dated) in the refrigerator for up to 3 weeks.

Curry Spice Blend
Makes approximately 1 cup

One of my favorite flavorings to have on hand, this delicious, Indian-inspired blend adds an exotic edge to most bean and vegetable dishes. These spices are used in Ayurveda cooking for their healing benefits, and are known for their immunity-building properties.

Ingredients:
- ¼ cup ground ginger
- ⅛ cup ground cumin
- ⅛ cup ground coriander
- ¼ cup ground turmeric
- 1 tablespoon cinnamon or sweet paprika

Simply blend the ground spices listed above and store in a glass jar (labeled and dated) in your spice cabinet for up to 8 months.

Basil Pesto
Makes 1½ cups

I've been making pesto from fresh herbs and various nut varieties since I was a kid, using whatever was in the garden and on hand, so after all these years it was really fun to encapsulate the options into a single recipe. This sauce is best made during summer months when fresh basil is in season. I make copious amounts and freeze in small containers for use well into the winter. It's delicious with pasta or in a stir-fry. Or spread it on a whole-wheat baguette, top with sliced tomato, and pop in the oven for a mouth-watering treat!

Ingredients:
- 2 packed cups fresh basil leaves (organic if possible)
- 3 cloves garlic; *or* 1½ teaspoons powdered or granulated garlic
- ½ cup olive oil
- ¼ cup pine nuts or walnuts
- 1 teaspoon salt

Combine all ingredients in a blender or food processor. If working with a blender, you may need to stop it intermittently and push the leaves down with a spatula before starting up again, to help pulverize them. Once all ingredients are incorporated into a thick, even consistency, turn off the blender and spoon the pesto into a serving bowl and use it within a day or two, or freeze in airtight containers (labeled and dated) for up to 2 months.

Seven-minute Marinara Sauce
2 to 4 servings

This is tastier alternative to jarred marinara sauce, and easy to pull together in a jiffy. Serve it with whole-grain pasta and cannellini beans for a simple, satisfying meal.

Ingredients:
- 1 tablespoon olive oil
- 1 medium onion, diced (approximately one cup)
- 1 teaspoon salt
- 2 to 3 cloves garlic, crushed (preferred); *or* 2 teaspoons powdered or granulated garlic
- 1 29-ounce (BPA-free) can diced tomatoes (Muir Glen is a favorite)

- 2 rounded tablespoons capers, including liquid;
  or 1 tablespoon Asian fish sauce
- 1 tablespoon Italian seasoning
- 1 teaspoon sugar or ½ teaspoon stevia
- 1 teaspoon crushed red pepper (optional)

Heat olive oil in a large sauté pan; add onion, garlic, Italian seasoning, and salt, and sauté for 5 minutes, adding liquid from diced tomatoes if more liquid is needed. When onions are translucent, add capers, tomatoes, and remaining ingredients. Bring to a simmer and it's ready to serve.

Nada Cheese Topping
Makes 1 cup

Full-flavored and zesty, this topping is a great dairy-free alternative to Parmesan cheese. Try adding a dash of it to salads, breads, and soups.

Ingredients:
- ½ cup nutritional yeast (a popular cheese substitute; available in the spice section of most health-food stores)
- ½ cup raw cashews or almonds
- 1 teaspoon salt
- ¼ cup sesame seeds

Combine all ingredients in a blender and pulverize until nuts are finally chopped. Store in the refrigerator for up to 4 months.

Cashew Cream
Makes ¾ cup

This rich and creamy dairy substitute is a cinch to make. The trick is to soak the cashews for a velvety finished texture. Add it to vegetable soups and stews to give them a rich, creamy texture, or blend with your favorite fruit and freeze for a lovely dessert.

Ingredients:
- ¾ cup raw cashews, soaked for at least 30 minutes (or up to 8 hours) in enough water just to cover them
- ½ teaspoon salt

Drain soaked cashews, reserving ¼ cup liquid. Add cashews and salt to a blender or food processor and puree until smooth, adding liquid as needed for blending, or until the mixture reaches your preferred consistency. It can be stored in the fridge for up to 5 days, or in the freezer for up to 2 months.

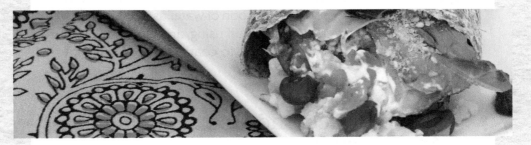

The Basics

On those days when you're caught without a plan (we all have them!) and the pressure's on to whip something up in a hurry, here are some easy, throw-together ideas for delicious, nutritious, one-dish meals.

Snappy Veggie Stir-fry
4 to 6 servings

More of a cooking method than a formal recipe, this dish invites you to use whatever you have on hand. Add a sauce (pre-made if possible), some tofu, and a grain—and you've got all your bases deliciously covered.

Ingredients:
- 1 tablespoon olive or coconut oil
- 2 to 3 cups of any of the following, coarsely chopped: carrots (peel on or off), cabbage, celery, onion (peeled), broccoli florets, cauliflower florets
- 1 cup extra-firm tofu, cut into 1-inch cubes (optional)
- 1 cup bean sprouts or sliced mushrooms (optional)
- 1 teaspoon salt
- ½ cup of any of the following sauces: Vegan Curry, Ginger Peanut, Cilantro Mint, or Basil Pesto (see pages 139, 202, 138, or 144 respectively)

Heat oil in a large saucepan on medium-high heat, add chopped vegetables and tofu, and stir-fry for 5 to 10 minutes, until tender. If mixture becomes dry, add a tablespoon of water as needed to prevent burning. Add mushrooms or sprouts if using, and sauté for 2 minutes longer. Mix in salt and sauce and stir to coat. Remove from heat and serve.

Simple Rice and Bean Bowls
Single serving suggestion

These are perfect make-ahead meals which can be easily adapted to include the ingredients you have on hand. I save a lot of money (and empty calories) by creating a version of this dish every day for lunch—this way I know in advance what I'm eating *and* I don't have to wait in line for takeout. Essentially, it's just the basics: a bean, a green, and a grain, put together into a single dish. The trick is to use your leftovers, which when combined as suggested come together in a flavorful new way. And no hassle required!

Ingredients:
- Cooked grains: 1 to 2 cups of your choice of rice, quinoa, or whatever you have left from last night's meal
- Topping ideas: 1 to 2 cups sautéed greens or some leftover bean salad, steamed veggies, or even a flavorful thick soup

To pack your lunch, just place your grains into a to-go container and layer with the topping of your choosing. Cover and refrigerate until ready to enjoy, warmed or as is.

For eating at home, place your grains along with 2 tablespoons of water in a saucepan over medium heat for 4 to 6 minutes. In a separate pan, heat or prepare your toppings. Layer heated grains with topping of choice into a bowl and serve.

Wrap and Roll!
1 serving

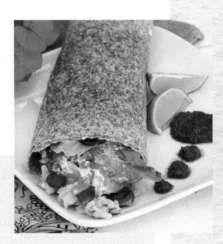

Wraps make a quick, healthy, and delicious lunch or dinner. They're also great for kids' lunches.

Ingredients:
- 1 whole-grain burrito-sized wrap
- The filling of your choice

Filling suggestions:
- Cover a thin layer of white bean dip with a mixture of fresh arugula leaves lightly tossed in balsamic vinegar, a few tablespoons of diced tomato, and a layer of thinly sliced cucumber
- Top ¼ cup hummus with chopped olives, chopped lettuce, shredded carrot, and some Tahini Vinaigrette (see page 143)
- Cover a layer of Red Pepper Cashew Spread (see page 135) with spinach leaves, sliced smoked tofu, and sliced avocado
- Drizzle a cup or two of mixed salad greens (or last night's leftover salad) with your favorite dressing

Prepare it burrito-style by piling ingredients in the center of the wrap, or spread everything evenly onto the surface and roll it up like you're rolling your yoga mat after a rejuvenating class. As always, feel free to experiment and invent your own favorites.

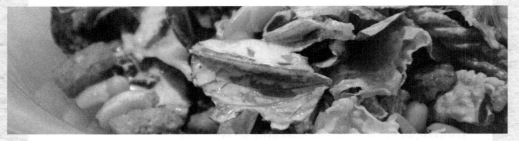

Hearty Salads

I'm a true salad lover. Even if the health benefits weren't so tremendous I'd probably still be a fan. I love that there are so many different salad options—there's sure to be something to tempt every palate. So enjoy your greens, stick with your standbys, and whenever the mood strikes you, try some of these delicious new blends.

Quinoa Tabouli
4 servings

A yummy high-protein take on a classic summer favorite. Best to enjoy when cucumbers are fresh and in season. I love using my mini food processer for chopping the herbs, which saves a lot of prep time; but chopping by hand is a great option, too. The quinoa may be prepared in advance for this dish, since it's served cold.

Ingredients:
- 1 large English cucumber, peeled and diced (2 to 3 cups)
- 1 cup quinoa
- ¼ cup black lentils
- ½ red onion, finely chopped
- 4 tablespoons olive oil
- ¼ cup lemon juice (fresh if available)
- ½ cup parsley, finely chopped (a mini food processor or spice grinder is helpful if available)
- 4 tablespoons mint, finely chopped (see above)
- 1 tomato (variety of your choice; approximately 1 cup), seeded and diced
- 1 teaspoon salt

Bring 3 cups of water to a boil in a saucepan. Add quinoa and black lentils, bring to simmering, then reduce heat to low; cover and cook for 20 to 25 minutes or until the water is absorbed. Remove from heat and allow quinoa mixture to cool. Mix in remaining ingredients and serve.

Orange, Fennel, and Kamut Salad
6 servings

Chewy, whole-grain kamut is making a comeback, and this savory flavor combination is a wonderful way to enjoy it. I prefer to soak my kamut for at least 8 hours or overnight before cooking, but it's not a must-do if you find yourself in a time crunch. Serve as a side dish or over some fresh arugula for a yummy main dish.

Ingredients:
- 1½ cups whole-grain kamut (soaked overnight if possible), rinsed and drained
- 2¾ cups water
- 1 cube or 1 teaspoon vegetable bouillon
- 1 large seedless orange, peeled, separated into sections, and sliced into ¼-inch pieces
- ½ cup dried, unsweetened cranberries
- 2 tablespoons olive oil
- 1 tablespoon balsamic vinegar
- 1 medium bulb fennel, finely chopped
- ½ cup scallions, chopped
- ¼ cup pecans or sunflower seeds, chopped
- ½ teaspoon salt
- Black pepper to taste

Place kamut in a saucepan with 2¾ cups water and salt. Bring to a boil, cover, and simmer for 50 to 60 minutes over low heat, until almost all the liquid is absorbed. Turn off the burner, but leave the pan on the stove. Add fennel and scallions to the pot, cover, and let sit for 5 minutes longer. Remove from heat and cool for 30 minutes, then add the remaining ingredients. Serve warm or at room temperature.

Harvest Salad
4 servings

Rice and veggies merge deliciously in this hearty, healthy salad. Since mung beans don't need to be soaked before cooking, it's easy to add some plant protein to this wonderfully textured dish without having to plan ahead.

Ingredients:
- 1 cup brown or black rice
- 1 cup mung beans
- 1 cup red cabbage, diced
- 2 medium carrots, diced (approximately 1 cup)
- 1 cup broccoli or cauliflower, chopped into small pieces
- 6 tablespoons Savory Sauce Blend (see page 141)

Optional:
- ½ cup smoked or teriyaki-style tofu, diced (or plain firm if unavailable)

In a large saucepan, bring 6 to 8 cups water to a simmer over medium-high heat. Add beans and simmer (just below boiling) until tender, for 1¼ hours. Remove from heat, drain, and rinse, then pour into a large salad bowl. Bring 2 cups of water and 1 cup of rice to a boil in a small saucepan. Reduce to a simmer, cover, and cook until rice is tender and liquid is absorbed, about 45 minutes. Turn off the heat, but leave pan on the stove. Stir in veggies and remaining ingredients, cover, and let stand for 10 minutes. Blend rice mixture in with mung beans and serve warm or at room temperature.

Zesty Five-bean Salad
12 servings

This salad is so scrumptious, I've been known to go on a tear and eat it for five days straight, which is why the recipe makes so much! Then I take a break for a month or two before I remember how good it is, and start all over again. Fortunately it's super-easy to make. The trick is in the unique bean mix and the al dente–style cooking. With the small bean varieties used in this dish you can get away with it, and the resulting texture is just unbeatable.

However, if you prefer your beans fully cooked, add 15 minutes to the cooking time recommended below. And if 12 servings is daunting or just plain crazy for you, simply divide the ingredients by two for a half-sized outcome.

Ingredients:
- 1 cup each: mung beans, adzuki beans, and whole green peas (if available), soaked in 12 cups of water overnight. (Don't worry if you don't have all three types of beans—just use what you have!)
- 3 carrots, diced (optional)
- ½ cup scallions, thinly sliced, or red onion, diced
- ½ cup parsley, chopped (a blender or mini food processor is perfect for this)
- 4 tablespoons olive oil
- ¼ cup balsamic vinegar
- 1 teaspoon powdered or granulated garlic
- 1 to 2 teaspoons salt
- 1 cup walnuts, chopped
- ¼ cup pitted dates, diced

Drain and rinse dry beans, then add to a large stockpot; fill with water to 6 inches over the top of the dry bean blend. Turn heat to medium-high and bring to a low boil, then reduce heat to simmer and cook for 1 to 1¼ hours. Drain and rinse, then return drained beans to pot. Add remaining ingredients, mix, and let cool. Serve at room temperature or chilled.

Basic Three-bean Salad
8 to10 servings

I've avoided including the more commonly known bean dishes among the Beanalicious recipes—unless they're just too good to leave out. This recipe is one of them. Ridiculously easy, it's also a total crowd-pleaser, which makes it the perfect potluck dish. Be sure to plan ahead, as the beans need to be soaked at least 8 hours before cooking.

Ingredients:

- 1 cup each: kidney beans, garbanzo beans, and navy beans
- 2 cups green beans, fresh or frozen (if using frozen, allow them to thaw)
- ¾ cup parsley, chopped (a blender or mini food processor is perfect for this)
- ⅓ cup balsamic vinegar
- ¼ to ⅓ cup olive oil (more oil gives it more flavor, but also more fat so choose accordingly)
- 1 teaspoon salt
- 1 teaspoon powdered or granulated garlic

To prepare beans from scratch, soak for at least 8 hours or overnight. Drain and rinse beans, then add to a large stockpot; fill with water to 6 inches over the top of the bean blend. Turn heat to medium-high and bring to a low boil, then reduce heat to simmer and cook for 1 to 1¼ hours. Place cooked beans in a large salad bowl and stir in green beans. Add remaining ingredients and mix well. This salad is even more delicious when you let it sit for at least an hour before serving. It's wonderful the next day, or refrigerated for up to one week, too.

Shitake Kale Salad
6 servings

A true power blend, this is one of my dietary staples. Admittedly you must be a kale lover to enjoy it, but many have been converted after giving this flavorful salad a try.

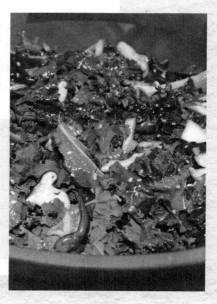

Ingredients:

- 4 to 6 cups kale, chopped or torn into bite-sized pieces
- 2 tablespoons sesame oil
- 6 to 8 shiitake mushrooms, thinly sliced
- ½ cup scallions, thinly sliced (use both white and green parts)

- ¼ cup Savory Sauce Blend (see page 141); *or* 2 tablespoons Bragg Liquid Aminos, 1 teaspoon Asian fish sauce (optional), and 2 tablespoons rice vinegar
- ½ teaspoon salt
- 2 tablespoons sesame seeds (toasted or untoasted)

Combine kale and sesame oil in a large salad bowl. Lightly toss, then "massage" the kale a bit with your fingers to slightly wilt it. Add remaining ingredients, toss, and serve.

Bean Sprout Salad
6 to 8 servings

Light and zesty, this refreshing dish is packed with nutrients and flavor. Sprout your own mungs, or buy them ready-sprouted for an extra-crunchy treat. Sunflower seeds or toasted slivered almonds can be substituted for peanuts to give you some further options. This salad takes a bit of chopping in the prep stage, but once you get through that part, it's a simple toss and serve away!

Ingredients:
- 2 cups mung bean sprouts
- 4 cups arugula, chopped
- 1 large daikon radish, finely chopped
- 2 bunches scallions, thinly sliced
- 1 teaspoon salt
- ½ cup peanuts, raw (skin off) or roasted, coarsely chopped
- 1 serrano chili pepper, stemmed and halved, seeds in or out depending on how hot you like it; the more seeds, the hotter it gets (optional)
- ½ cup Cilantro Mint Sauce (see page 138)

Prep the sprouts, arugula, radish, and scallions, then place into a salad bowl, add salt, and toss to blend. Add the Cilantro Mint Sauce, chili pepper (if using), and peanuts; toss to thoroughly combine. Serve immediately.

Crunchy Cashew Fennel Slaw

8 servings

This simple salad is always a crowd-pleaser. In the off chance there are leftovers, it's even better enjoyed the following day (or two!).

Ingredients:
- 1 large carrot, shredded or thinly sliced into matchstick-shaped pieces
- 3 to 4 cups cabbage, shredded or finely chopped
- 1 large fennel bulb, thinly sliced
- ¼ cup Cilantro Mint Sauce (see page 138)
- 1 teaspoon powdered or granulated garlic
- 3 tablespoons rice vinegar
- 1 teaspoon salt
- ¼ cup Thai-spiced cashews, chopped (use plain roasted if unavailable)

Combine all ingredients in large salad bowl, then let the spices blend for at least 30 minutes before serving. Even better when left to marinate, store this crunchy salad in the fridge for up to 3 days.

Lemon Cumin Rice Salad

6 to 8 servings

Simple and refreshing, this flavorful salad is high in nutrients, too. Unlike most bean salads, you'll want to use this within the first day or two of preparation before the rice dries out.

Ingredients:
- 1 cup short- or medium-grain brown rice
- 3½ cups water
- 1 cup black lentils
- ½ cup parsley, chopped (use a blender or mini food processor for easy prepping)

- 1 large green pepper, seeded and diced
- ⅓ cup Lemon Cumin Dressing (see page 141)
- Additional salt to taste

Bring water to a boil in a medium-sized saucepan. Add rice and return just briefly to simmer. Cover and reduce heat. Cook for 20 minutes and add lentils. Cover and cook for 25 to 30 minutes longer, until water is absorbed. Let sit covered for 5 to 10 minutes longer, then remove from heat and stir in remaining ingredients. Let marinate for at least 30 minutes, otherwise refrigerate for up to 8 hours before serving, since the flavors intensify the longer it sits. Serve at room temperature.

White Bean Caesar Salad
4 to 6 servings

This is an egg-free Caesar salad, very tasty and a bit healthier than the traditional version. A kid favorite in our house for sure.

Ingredients:
- ½ cup raw cashews, soaked in water for at least 30 minute
- ¼ cup soaking water from cashews
- 1 tablespoon olive oil
- ¼ cup soy, rice, or almond milk
- 3 tablespoons lemon juice (fresh if available)
- 1 tablespoon spicy brown mustard
- 1 clove garlic; *or* 1 teaspoon powdered or granulated garlic
- 1 teaspoon Worcestershire sauce or Bragg Liquid Aminos
- ¾ teaspoon salt (to taste)
- 1 rounded tablespoon jarred capers or 2 teaspoons Asian fish sauce
- 2 cups small white beans, precooked
- 1 head romaine lettuce (6 to 8 cups), cut into bite-sized pieces
- Whole-wheat garlic croutons (homemade or a good store brand)
- Ground pepper to taste

To prepare beans from scratch, soak for at least 8 hours or overnight. Drain and rinse, then add them to a large stockpot and fill with water so it covers the beans by at least 6 inches. Turn heat to medium-high and bring to a low boil, then reduce heat to simmer and cook for 1½ to 2 hours until tender. Drain and rinse in cold water to cool.

Add the first 10 ingredients (cashews to capers/fish sauce) to a blender. Puree until smooth. Add the lettuce to a large serving bowl and toss with dressing and beans. Season with pepper, add croutons, and serve.

Glorious Green Garbanzo Bean Salad
6 to 8 servings

Much as I love my garbanzo beans, when used in a salad I feel these hearty nuggets are best paired with veggies to temper their density. The aromatic herbs make this savory salad as flavorful as it is satisfying.

Ingredients:
- 4 cups garbanzo beans, precooked (use hot or cool)
- 1 small red onion, peeled and finely chopped (about ½ cup)
- 3 large stalks celery, diced (about 1 cup)
- 1 red or green pepper, seeded and diced
- ¼ cup olive oil
- ¼ cup balsamic vinegar
- ½ cup parsley, finely chopped (a mini food processor or spice blender is perfect for this)
- 1 tablespoon ground cumin
- 1½ teaspoons salt

To prepare beans from scratch, soak for at least 8 hours or overnight. Drain and rinse, then add to a large stockpot and fill with water to cover beans by at least 6 inches. Turn heat to medium-high and bring to a low boil, then reduce heat to simmer and cook for 1½ to 2½ hours. Drain and rinse.

Combine all ingredients. This dish is best when allowed to marinate at least 30 minutes prior to serving. Like many bean salads, it's even better the next day. Serve plain or over a bed of arugula for a delicious one-dish meal.

Thai Cabbage Salad
8 servings

This simple coleslaw-style salad tantalizes with a light and zesty finish. It's so easy to prepare, I frequently mix one together as a last-minute salad option, since I always have cabbage and carrots on hand and all it requires is a bit of chopping.

Ingredients:
- 1 large carrot, shredded (by hand or in a mini food processor), or thinly sliced into matchstick-shaped pieces
- 3 to 4 cups cabbage, shredded or finely chopped
- ½ cup scallions, finely chopped
- ½ cup cilantro, finely chopped (a mini food processor is recommended if you have one available)
- ¼ cup Savory Sauce Blend (see page 141); *or* 2 tablespoons Bragg Liquid Aminos, 4 tablespoons rice vinegar, and 1 to 2 teaspoons Asian fish sauce
- 2 tablespoons sesame oil
- ¼ cup roasted peanuts, chopped

Combine all ingredients in large salad bowl. Best to let the spices blend for at least 30 minutes before serving.

Corn and Black Bean Salad
8 to 10 servings

This simple salad is great for a picnic or potluck, or nice for an easy summer dinner at home. If you cook your beans right before making this dish, the heat will slightly steam the onion and celery—

which I like. But completely raw, crisp veggies are delicious, too. Just be sure to finely chop, which is where a mini food processor really comes in handy.

Ingredients:
- 4 cups black beans, precooked, hot or cool
- 2 cups fresh or frozen corn
- ¾ cup celery, finely chopped
- ¾ cup red onion, finely chopped
- ¼ cup cilantro, finely chopped (a mini food processor is recommended if available)
- 2 teaspoons chili powder
- 4 tablespoons olive oil
- 4 tablespoons lime juice (fresh if available)
- 2 teaspoons salt
- ¼ cup pine nuts (optional)

To prepare dried beans from scratch, soak for at least 8 hours or overnight. Drain and rinse, then add to a large stockpot and fill with water to cover the beans by at least 6 inches. Turn heat to medium-high and bring to a low boil, then reduce heat to simmer and cook for 1 to 1¼ hours.

Strain beans and add to a large mixing bowl with celery and onion. Toss and let sit for 10 to 15 minutes before adding remaining ingredients; continue to let cool, then serve.

If you're using leftover beans: combine all ingredients and let sit at room temperature for at least an hour before serving. This dish is even better prepared a day ahead.

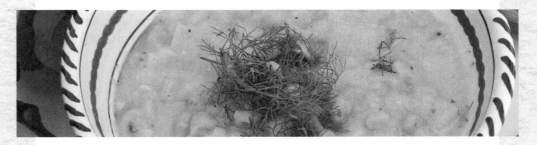

Soups and Stews

One-pot meals are a cook's delight, especially when time is of the essence. When it comes to soups and stews, I love the flexibility I have. Improvisation is welcome! No carrots? Substitute parsnips, or celery, or whatever you have on hand. There are no wrong answers when it comes to fresh veggies! So fill your pot with lots of healthy, nutritious goodness and let your creative juices flow.

Black Bean Soup
6 servings

Hearty, filling, and delicious, this soup is a staple in our house. Vary the vegetables, herbs, and consistency to work with the seasons: thinner and abundant in tomato and fresh herbs for summer, thick and hearty with zestier spices for fall. I love to make a big pot, enjoy leftovers for lunch, and still have enough left for a second meal.

Ingredients:
- 4 cups dried black beans, precooked
- 2 tablespoons coconut oil
- 1 large or two small onions, chopped (about 2 cups)
- 3 stalks celery, chopped (optional)
- 1 tablespoon ground cumin
- 1 tablespoon powdered or granulated garlic
- 6 to 8 cups vegetable broth (*or* 3 to 4 teaspoons bouillon *or* 3 to 4 bouillon cubes, dissolved in 6 to 8 cups of water)
- Salt and pepper to taste

- Optional garnish: finely diced tomato or chopped cilantro (a mini food processor makes the prep work of chopping the cilantro very easy)

To prepare beans from scratch, soak for at least 8 hours or overnight. Drain and rinse after soaking, then add to a large stockpot and fill with water to cover the beans by at least 6 inches. Turn heat to medium-high and bring to a low boil, then reduce heat to simmer and cook for 1 to 1¼ hours.

In a large stockpot, sauté the onion, celery, and cumin in coconut oil on medium-high heat until onions are translucent, about 5 minutes. Stir in garlic, then add half of the cooked beans, salt, and vegetable broth and bring to a simmer. Remove from heat and let the mixture cool down enough to work with. Using either a hand or standing blender, blend the soup in the pot or add to a blender and puree.

Once the soup is pureed, add the rest of the beans and broth to it in the pot and heat to desired temperature to serve. Garnish with topping of choice.

Simple Bean and Green Soup
8 servings

True vegetarian soul food, this simple soup satisfies even the heartiest of eaters. This recipe makes an ample batch, enough to reheat and serve again later in the week or to place in the freezer for a fast future meal. Serve it with a salad and some crusty whole-grain bread for a wonderfully rounded meal.

Ingredients:
- 1 tablespoon olive oil
- 1 large bulb or 1 cup fennel, chopped (use celery if fennel is unavailable)
- 1 large onion, chopped
- 1 to 2 teaspoons salt (less if using Asian fish sauce)
- 8 cups vegetable broth (or dissolve 6 cubes or teaspoons

vegetable bouillon in 8 cups of water)
- 4 cups white (navy) beans, precooked
- 1 to 2 bunches escarole or collard greens, stems removed, coarsely chopped (about 4 cups)
- ¼ cup pesto, jarred or homemade (see page 144)
- Salt and pepper to taste

Optional:
- 2 tablespoons Asian fish sauce
- ½ cup Nada Cheese Topping (see page 146) or grated Parmesan cheese

To prepare beans from scratch, soak for at least 8 hours or overnight. Drain and rinse after soaking, then add to a large stockpot and fill with water to cover the beans by at least 6 inches. Turn heat to medium-high and bring to a low boil, then reduce heat to simmer and cook for 1½ hours.

Heat the oil in a large pot on medium-high. Add fennel, onion, salt, and fish sauce (if using) and cook for 5 minutes, until vegetables begin to brown. Add the beans, kale, and broth (or water and bouillon). Cover and bring to a boil, then reduce heat and simmer until greens are tender, 4 to 5 minutes. Remove from heat and stir in the pesto, then let sit for 1 hour before serving.

Minestrone Soup
8 to 12 servings

An Italian classic as well as a healthy favorite, minestrone soup is real comfort food. This simple version is lovely paired with a green salad and crusty whole-grain bread for a warm and wonderful meal.

Ingredients:
- 1 tablespoon olive oil
- 1 medium onion, diced
- 1 cup green beans, chopped into ½-inch pieces
- 1 large fennel bulb or 4 celery stalks, diced

- 3 carrots, diced
- 2 cups cannellini or garbanzo beans, precooked
- 3 vegetable bouillon cubes dissolved in 4 cups of water
- 3 to 4 cups fresh tomatoes, diced, or a similar amount of BPA-free canned or jarred
- 1½ teaspoons powdered or granulated garlic; *or* 2 cloves garlic, crushed
- 2 teaspoons dried Italian seasoning (parsley, basil, and oregano, or equivalent amounts of whatever you have on hand)
- 1 to 2 teaspoons salt (to taste)
- Fresh ground black pepper to taste
- ½ to 1 cup whole-grain or quinoa pasta

Note: See the Bean Soaking and Cooking Chart on page 116 for bean preparation instructions.

In a large saucepot, sauté cut vegetables, garlic, salt, and seasoning in oil over medium-high heat until slightly softened, 10 to 15 minutes. Add tomatoes and cook for 2 minutes longer. Add water and beans, and bring the soup to a low simmer. Cover and continue to cook at a low simmer for 30 minutes, stirring occasionally. Increase the temperature slightly, then add pasta and cook 15 to 20 minutes longer until cooked through according to directions or to taste.

Savory Ginger Carrot Soup
6 servings

This lively soup is a wellness bonanza, with ginger and spices that both enhance the flavor and give your immune system an extra boost. The ginger is potent, so adjust according to your preference. Enjoy it hot, poured over a warm bowl of rice or quinoa as a nourishing meal, or hold the beans and serve it cold for a light and refreshing summer bisque.

Ingredients:
- 1 onion, peeled and chopped
- 5½ cups water
- 4 cups carrots (peel on is fine), coarsely chopped
- ½- to 1-inch piece of fresh ginger, unpeeled
- 3 cubes or teaspoons vegetable bouillon
- ½ teaspoon ground cinnamon
- 1 teaspoon ground cumin
- 1 tablespoon honey or ½ teaspoon stevia
- ½ to 1 teaspoon salt
- 2 cups cannellini beans, precooked
- ½ cup roasted sunflower seeds for topping (optional)

To prepare beans from scratch, soak for at least 8 hours or overnight. Drain and rinse after soaking, then add to a large stockpot and fill with water to cover the beans by at least 6 inches. Turn heat to medium-high and bring to a low boil, then reduce heat to simmer and cook for 1½ to 2 hours. Drain and rinse.

Add the onion, carrots, and ginger to a large saucepan with ½ to 1 cup water (about ½ inch) and simmer, covered, over medium heat until soft and translucent, 10 to 12 minutes. Remove pan from heat and let stand, covered, for 5 minutes longer. Pour the mixture into a blender or food processor with the remaining ingredients, except for the beans. Puree until soup is smooth and creamy, then pour mixture back into pan, add beans, and reheat to serve. Top with sunflower seeds if desired.

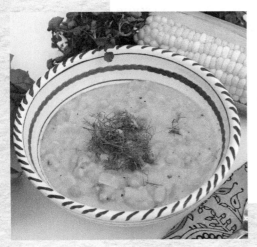

Corn Chowder
4 servings

This creamy veggie chowder conjures up visions of summers on the Rhode Island coast, where "chowdah," as it's commonly pronounced, is a staple on every menu. This flavorful soup is quick, easy, and delicious, with or without the seafood (here not included).

Ingredients:

- 1 onion, very coarsely chopped
- 2 large leeks (whites only), chopped
- 1 large or 2 small fennel bulbs, coarsely chopped (about 1 cup)
- 1½ cup water (use the liquid from the steamed veggies and bring to final volume)
- 1½ cups rice milk
- 1 teaspoon salt
- 1 clove garlic; *or* 1 teaspoon powdered or granulated garlic
- 1 teaspoon capers
- 1 cup corn (fresh or frozen)
- 1 cup cooked navy or white beans, precooked
- Ground black pepper to taste

To prepare beans from scratch, soak for at least 8 hours or overnight. Drain and rinse after soaking, then add to a large stockpot and fill with water to cover the beans by at least 6 inches. Turn heat to medium-high and bring to a low boil, then reduce heat to simmer and cook for 1½ to 2 hours. Drain and rinse.

Add the onion, leeks, and fennel to a large saucepan with ½ to 1 cup water (about ½ inch) and simmer, covered, over medium heat until soft and translucent, 8 to 10 minutes. Remove pan from heat and let stand, covered, for 5 minutes longer. Pour the mixture into the blender with enough additional water to equal 1½ cups total. Add rice milk, seasonings, and capers; blend until smooth. Pour soup back into saucepan and add corn and white beans.

Nonvegetarians in the spirit of New England might cook in some fresh clams or sustainably harvested scallops, but chopped tempeh bacon makes a delicious addition, too.

Curried Sweet Potato and Lentil Soup

6 to 8 servings

This yummy dish is supercharged with healthy ingredients, and a cinch to make, despite the exotic flavor combinations. Bountiful enough to go solo, or serve with some brown rice on the side and a simple green salad topped with some Lemon Cumin Dressing (see page 141) for a flavorful multicourse meal.

Ingredients:

- 1 medium onion, peeled and coarsely chopped
- 1 large sweet potato, peeled, cut lengthwise then again into ½- to 1-inch pieces
- 1 apple, peeled, cored, and coarsely chopped
- 4 to 5 cups vegetable broth; *or* equivalent amount of water and 3 teaspoons or cubes of vegetable bouillon
- 1 cup lentils, variety of your choice
- 1 teaspoon Curry Spice Blend (see page 144)
- ½ cup Vegan Curry Sauce (see page 139) or Cashew Cream (see page 146)
- 1 tablespoon honey or stevia
- 1 teaspoon lemon pepper blend (optional)
- 1 teaspoon salt (or to taste)

Add 1 inch of water to a large pot and bring to a simmer. Add sweet potato and cover. Cook for 10 minutes, then add onion and cook for 5 minutes longer. Add the apple and turn off the heat, but leave the pot on the stove, covered, for 5 minutes longer. Pour the mixture into a blender with 2 cups of water and puree, then return the soup to the pan. Add remaining water and vegetable bouillon. Stir in remaining ingredients and bring to a simmer. Cook for 20 to 35 minutes longer, depending on the lentil variety you choose (red and yellow cook more quickly). Remove from heat and serve.

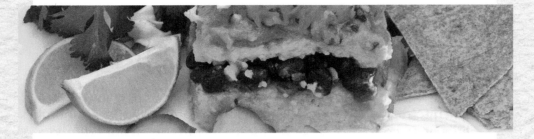

Entrees

Of course these recipes were selected for ease of use, availability of ingredients, and health benefits, but the most important criterion is *always* taste. And do keep in mind the Beanalicious penchant for flexibility in food preparation: substitute freely, measure loosely, and add your personal touch whenever the mood strikes you!

Fennel, White Bean, and Collard Green Sauté

4 servings

This lovely, appetizing dish is easy to prepare. Boiling the fennel stalks and greens in water until the liquid becomes concentrated, is a marvelous way to make your own aromatic consommé in one simple step. Serve this nourishing dish with wild rice or crusty whole-grain bread.

Ingredients:
- 1 whole fennel bulb, stalks and greens included
- 6 cups water
- 1 tablespoon olive oil
- 2 cups navy or cannellini beans, precooked
- 3 cups collard greens, stems removed, sliced into thin ribbons
- 2 cloves garlic; *or* 1 teaspoon powdered or granulated garlic
- 1 teaspoon salt
- 1 teaspoon dried oregano or Italian seasoning blend

Note: See the Bean Soaking and Cooking Chart on page 116 for bean preparation instructions.

To make consommé: remove stalks and greens from fennel bulb, rinse thoroughly, and add them to a large saucepan with 6 cups of water. Bring to a simmer over medium heat, cover, and cook down for about 30 minutes. In the meantime, chop fennel bulb into inch-long, very thin slices.

When consommé is reduced to 2 to 3 cups, remove from heat, and pour the consommé liquid only into a glass jar. Set aside. Toss out the remaining cooked fennel.

Add olive oil to the saucepan, and return to medium heat. Add chopped fennel and sauté over medium-high heat for 5 minutes. Add ¼ cup of consommé and simmer on medium-low for 5 more minutes, then repeat. Add ¼ cup more consommé, collard greens, and remaining seasonings and cook for 5 to 8 minutes longer, until greens are tender. Stir in beans and serve warm or hot. Label, date, and store remaining consommé in the fridge for up to 1 week, or freeze for up to 3 months.

Lentil Stuffed Peppers
4 servings

A bit more complex than most Beanalicious recipes, these savory stuffed peppers are a flavorful treat. Spice them up with some hot sauce or red pepper flakes if that's your preference, or skip the peppers altogether and serve the lentil stuffing as a tasty side dish.

Ingredients:
- 4 whole red or green peppers, tops sliced off and seeds removed
- 2 cups black lentils
- 1 tablespoon coconut oil
- 1 large onion, finely chopped
- 1 small handful parsley (about ¼ cup), finely chopped (a spice blender or mini food processor works great for this)

- 2 cups crimini, Portobello, or white mushrooms, chopped
- ¼ cup walnuts, finely chopped (by hand or in blender)
- 1 teaspoon or 1 cube vegetable bouillon dissolved in ¼ cup water
- 1 clove garlic; *or* ½ teaspoon powdered or granulated garlic
- 2 tablespoons Bragg Liquid Aminos
- ½ teaspoon salt
- 1 tablespoon chili powder
- 1 teaspoon red chili pepper flakes (optional)

Add 2 cups lentils to at least 8 cups boiling water and cook for 30 minutes until tender.

To prepare the peppers, preheat oven to 375°. Place the peppers cut side down on a metal cookie sheet and bake for 8 minutes until softened.

To make the stuffing, heat coconut oil in a large sauté pan over medium-high heat. Add onions and sauté for 3 minutes. Add mushrooms, parsley, Bragg Liquid Aminos, and salt, then sauté for 3 to 5 minutes longer until onion is translucent. Add water and garlic, then remove from heat and add lentils, walnuts, and chili powder. Finish with red pepper flakes if using.

Place stuffing into the partially cooked peppers and return to the oven. Bake for 15 to 20 minutes until tops begin to brown. Remove from the oven, let stand for at least 10 minutes, and serve.

Sicilian Garbanzo Marinara
4 servings as a main dish or 8 servings as a side dish

This flavorful, protein-rich stew is easy to make and wonderful served with hearty rice or whole-grain pasta, mixed together salad-like fashion, but it works nicely over polenta as well. I love using sprouted garbanzo beans for the crunchier texture, but unsprouted and cooked are equally delicious.

Ingredients:
- 3 cups garbanzo beans, precooked
- 1 medium onion, chopped (about 1 cup)

- 1 small red pepper, chopped
- 1 tablespoon olive oil
- ¼ cup water or vegetable broth (bouillon is fine)
- 1 15-ounce jar prepared garlic-and-basil-flavored marinara sauce; *or* 2 cups Seven-minute Marinara Sauce (see page 145)

To prepare beans from scratch, soak for at least 8 hours or overnight. Drain and rinse, then add the beans to a large stockpot and fill with water to cover the beans by at least 6 inches. Turn heat to medium-high and bring to a low boil, then reduce heat to simmer and cook for 1½ to 2½ hours. Drain and rinse.

In medium or large sauté pan, sauté onions and peppers in oil for 5 minutes or until translucent. If using diced tomato mixture, add all remaining ingredients and sauté for 2 minutes longer. If using prepared marinara, stir it in until heated through, then serve.

Betty's Bean Burritos
6 servings

Whip these up using leftover beans and rice for an easy dinner or satisfying lunch. I like to add shredded cabbage for an extra dash of green; as always, have fun creating your own version!

Ingredients:
- 2 cups cooked kidney beans, precooked
- 2 cups brown rice, precooked
- ½ to 1 teaspoon salt, to taste
- 6 whole-grain tortillas
- 1½ cups shredded cheese, vegan or dairy
- 1 ripe avocado, peeled and chopped
- 1½ cups salsa (jarred is fine; choose your preference, from mild to hot)

Optional:
- ½ cup olives
- 1 cup cabbage, shredded
- 1 cup smoked tofu, diced

Heat beans and rice separately by placing into a saucepan, adding ½ inch of water, and warming over medium heat, covered, for 2 to 3 minutes. If beans are unseasoned, stir in salt before serving.

Warm your tortillas by wrapping a stack of 6 tortillas in aluminum foil and place in a preheated 350° oven until heated through, 15 to 20 minutes.

Layer each warm tortilla with beans and rice and any other fillings you choose, spreading evenly in a line down the center. Top with cheese and salsa, tuck in the ends to keep the goodness in, roll up, and enjoy.

Mediterranean Kale and Bean Sauté
2 to 4 servings

This flavorful green sauté has a lovely Mediterranean-style flair, especially when served with Kalamata olives and chopped tomato. Substitute dairy cheese for sliced olives for a non-vegan version. Serve with a side of hearty grain or pasta for a satisfying meal.

Ingredients:
- 1 large head of curly kale or collard greens, coarsely chopped (4 to 6 cups)
- 2 tablespoons olive oil
- 1 red onion, sliced
- 1 teaspoon powdered or granulated garlic; *or* 2 cloves garlic, crushed
- 1 teaspoon dried Italian herb blend, dried basil, or dried oregano
- ½ to 1 teaspoon salt (to taste)
- 2 to 4 tablespoons water
- 1½ cups garbanzo or navy beans, precooked
- ¼ cup Nada Cheese Topping (see page 146) or ½ cup shredded Parmesan cheese

Optional:
- ¼ cup Kalamata olives, sliced
- 1 tomato, finely chopped

Note: See the Bean Soaking and Cooking Chart on page 116 for bean preparation instructions.

In a large sauté pan, heat oil and add onion, then cook for 2 minutes. Add chopped kale and stir-fry for 3 minutes longer. Add seasonings (garlic, salt, and herbs), plus ½ of the water (2 tablespoons), cover, and cook on low for 10 minutes. Stir halfway through and add more water if needed to prevent searing. Turn off the heat and stir in beans, cover, and let sit for at least 5 minutes more. Add remaining ingredients just before serving.

Curried Chickpeas and Potatoes
6 servings

This savory dish is delicious paired with brown rice and finished with a cool green or cucumber salad for a hearty one-pot, meat-free meal. Add chopped tofu for an extra protein punch.

Ingredients:
- 2 tablespoons coconut oil
- 2 large onions, diced
- 1 green pepper, seeded and diced
- 3 medium potatoes, peeled and cut into small (½-inch) cubes
- 1 15-ounce jar of BPA-free canned crushed tomatoes (Muir Glen is my favorite)
- 2 cups garbanzo beans, precooked
- 3 teaspoons Curry Spice Blend (see page 144)
- 1 teaspoon salt
- ½ to ¾ cup water

Optional:
- ¼ cup golden raisins
- 1 cup firm tofu (sprouted or smoked), chopped

To prepare beans from scratch, soak for at least 8 hours or overnight. Drain and rinse beans, then add to a large stockpot and fill with water to cover the beans by at least 6 inches. Turn heat to medium-high and bring to a low boil, then reduce heat to simmer and cook for 1½ to 2½ hours. Drain and rinse.

Add oil, potatoes, green pepper, onions, and ¼ cup water to a large sauté pan. Cover and cook over high heat for 5 to 7 minutes, stirring frequently, until onions become translucent. Add tomato sauce, beans, spices, and salt; cover and simmer for 25 to 35 minutes, stirring occasionally, until potatoes are tender. Add water, ¼ cup at a time, if mixture becomes dry during cooking. Add any optional ingredients and let stand, covered, for at least 5 minutes before serving.

North African Date Tangine
6 servings

Tangine is a North African word for both a special type of ceramic cookware and the succulent stew that's traditionally cooked inside. The exotic spices make this dish as fragrant as it is delicious.

Ingredients:
- 1 tablespoon coconut oil
- 2 large onions, diced
- 3 cloves garlic, crushed; *or* 2 teaspoons powdered or granulated garlic
- 2 teaspoons Curry Spice Blend (see page 144)
- ½ teaspoon cinnamon
- 3 cups garbanzo beans, precooked
- 2 cups jarred or 1 15-ounce can BPA-free crushed tomatoes (Muir Glen is my favorite)
- 2 cups whole-wheat couscous
- ¾ cup dates, pitted and cut into quarters

- Juice of 1 large lemon
- ½ cup cilantro, chopped (a mini food processor is recommended, if available)
- 1 teaspoon salt

To prepare beans from scratch, soak for at least 8 hours or overnight. Drain and rinse beans, then add to a large stockpot and fill with water to cover the beans by at least 6 inches. Turn heat to medium-high and bring to a low boil, then reduce heat to simmer and cook for 1½ to 2½ hours. Drain and rinse.

Sauté onion in oil in medium saucepan, stirring often, until it begins to brown, 6 to 8 minutes. Add garlic and Curry Spice Blend and sauté for 1 minute longer. Add tomato, garbanzo beans, and ¼ cup water. Cover and cook for 10 minutes longer.

In the meantime, prepare couscous by bringing 4 cups of water to a simmer in medium saucepan. Add couscous and return to boil, remove from heat, cover, and let stand for 5 minutes. Add dates, salt, and lemon juice to the tangine, stirring thoroughly. Serve over couscous.

Smoky Jo's Pinto Bean Sauté
4 servings

Crushed coriander seeds add the sensuous flavor to this tantalizing bean sauté, and don't forget the smoky marinated tempeh for a hearty kick. Serve over brown rice for a simple, delicious meal.

Ingredients:
- 2 cups pinto beans, precooked until soft
- 1 onion, peeled and chopped
- 1 tablespoon olive oil
- 1 clove garlic; *or* ½ teaspoon powdered or granulated garlic
- 1 teaspoon coriander seeds
- ½ teaspoon salt
- 1 teaspoon or 1 cube vegetable bouillon dissolved in ½ cup water

- 2 to 3 ounces marinated tempeh bacon (if available) or smoked tempeh, chopped
- ½ cup tomato sauce (jarred or BPA-free canned); or 1 large tomato, diced (seeds discarded)

To prepare beans from scratch, soak for at least 8 hours or overnight. Drain and rinse beans, then add to a large stockpot and fill with water to cover the beans by at least 6 inches. Turn heat to medium-high and bring to a low boil, then reduce heat to simmer and cook for 2 to 2¼ hours. Drain and rinse.

In a large, dry skillet, toast coriander seeds on medium heat, shaking to turn now and then, until fragrant, about 5 minutes. Cool slightly and crush by hand or toss in a spice or coffee grinder to coarsely chop. (If you go for the grinder, the lasting flavor is nice in coffee, too.)

Add olive oil and onion to the same skillet and sauté over low heat, about 5 to 8 minutes. Once translucent, add ¼ cup of veggie broth and cover. Raise the heat to medium/medium-high to simmer, and let cook for 5 to 8 minutes longer until most liquid is absorbed and onions are very soft. Add beans, garlic, coriander, and salt; cook, covered, for 5 minutes longer until most liquid is absorbed. Stir in tomato sauce and bacon. Cover pan and turn off heat, but leave the pan on the stove. Let stand for 5 minutes and serve over rice.

Sweet Potato and White Bean Chili
8 to 12 servings

Simple soul food never tasted so good. Toss up a big salad to serve on the side and your hearty, wholesome meal is complete.

Ingredients:
- 7 cups cannellini beans, precooked
- 2 large sweet potatoes, peeled and cubed (about 4 cups)
- 3 cubes or teaspoons vegetable bouillon cubes
- 2 tablespoons olive oil
- 1 large onion, chopped
- 1 tablespoon Curry Spice Blend (see page 144)

- 1 teaspoon salt
- 1 to 2 tablespoons chili powder (to taste)
- 1 tablespoon maple syrup (optional)
- 6 ounces smoke-flavored tofu or tempeh, diced (optional)

Soak beans overnight in a large stockpot. Drain beans and return to pot, then add enough water to cover beans by about 6 inches. Bring to simmer, then lower the temperature and cook on low heat for 1 hour; add potatoes and simmer for 30 to 45 minutes longer, until tender. In the meantime, place a sauté pan on medium heat, add olive oil, and sauté onion for 5 minutes, until translucent. Add seasoning, salt, and syrup (if using). Once beans are cooked, remove excess liquid with a ladle until the liquid is level with the beans and potatoes. Lightly mash the soup in the pot with a potato masher, then add the onion mixture and tofu or tempeh if using; cover and simmer for 15 minutes longer. Serve hot.

Pasta with Cannellini Beans and Arugula

4 servings

Arugula may be best known for bringing some spice to a fresh green salad, but this hearty green holds up well to heat for an alternative preparation style. Here it's paired with creamy cannellini beans for a zippy flavor combination. If arugula is out of season, spinach or chard leaves also work well in this dish.

Ingredients:
- 1 package whole-grain or quinoa pasta (12 to 16 ounces)
- 1 8.5-ounce jar sun-dried tomatoes in oil, drained and diced
- 1 head fresh arugula, coarsely chopped
- 1 cup cannellini beans, precooked
- ½ cup walnuts, chopped
- 1 tablespoon dried basil
- 1 teaspoon powdered or granulated garlic; *or* 2 cloves garlic, crushed

- 1 tablespoon olive oil
- ½ teaspoon salt
- ¼ cup shaved Parmesan cheese or 1 tablespoon Nada Cheese Topping (see page 146)

To prepare beans from scratch, soak for at least 8 hours or overnight. Drain and rinse beans, then add to a large stockpot and fill with water to cover the beans by at least 6 inches. Turn heat to medium-high and bring to a low boil, then reduce heat to simmer and cook for 1½ to 2 hours. Drain and rinse.

Cook pasta according to instructions on the package. Drain pasta, reserving ¼ cup of cooking liquid to use in the sauce. In a large skillet, sauté the arugula in olive oil, add seasonings, and cook until wilted, 2 to 4 minutes. Add sun-dried tomatoes, beans, and walnuts; stir until heated through. Add sauce to pasta and toss, adding some of the reserved cooking liquid if needed. Sprinkle with grated Parmesan cheese or Nada Cheese Topping and serve.

Mexican Caponata
4 servings

This zesty and flavorful ragout—a fancy word for "stew"—with its south-of-the-border flair will warm you when the leaves begin to change. Make it while late summer's eggplant and peppers are still abundant. Or take advantage of summer's bounty and serve it at room temperature during the warmer months. Delicious over rice or with a crusty whole-grain bread.

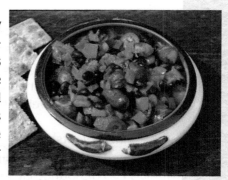

Ingredients:
- 1 tablespoon coconut oil
- 1 pound Italian or Asian eggplant, unpeeled, cut into ½-inch cubes
- 1 medium red onion, coarsely chopped

- 1 medium red pepper, diced
- ¼ cup cilantro, chopped (a mini food processor or spice grinder is helpful, if available)
- ½ cup salsa (you can use Basic Salsa, featured on page 134; jarred is fine also—choose your preference, from mild to hot)
- 1 cup black beans, precooked
- ½ to 1 teaspoon salt

To prepare beans from scratch, soak for at least 8 hours or overnight. Drain and rinse beans, then add to a large stockpot and fill with water to cover the beans by at least 6 inches. Turn heat to medium-high and bring to a low boil, then reduce heat to simmer and cook for 1½ to 2 hours. Drain and rinse.

Heat oil in a large saucepan on medium heat, then add eggplant, onion, and red pepper. Sauté until eggplant is cooked through and onion is translucent, 5 to 10 minutes. Turn off heat and mix in cilantro. Let the caponata stand for 10 minutes to blend, then add salsa, beans, and salt. Serve at room temperature with tortilla chips, rice, barley, or bread.

Easy Beanie Chili
10 servings

Nothing warms you up from the inside quite like homemade chili. This dish is so rich and hearty, you'll never miss the meat. It's easy to prepare, too, and makes great leftovers (and also freezes well). Feel free to mix different beans—black with pinto and kidney, or any combination you like. Serve with a side salad and a slice of corn bread for an easy meal.

Ingredients:
- 4 cups dried black beans, kidney beans, and/or pinto beans in any combination
- 2 large onions, chopped
- 1 tablespoon olive oil
- 2 cups tomato sauce (jarred or BPA-free canned)

- 4 cups bean cooking broth; *or* 4 cubes or teaspoons vegetable bouillon and 4 cups water
- 2 cups salsa (you can use Basic Salsa, featured on page 134; jarred is fine also—choose your preference, from mild to hot)
- 1 tablespoon chili powder
- Salt to taste
- 1 cup nondairy cheese or organic Monterey Jack cheese, shredded (optional)

To prepare beans from scratch, soak for at least 8 hours or overnight. Drain and rinse beans, then add to a large stockpot and fill with water to cover the beans by at least 6 inches. Turn heat to medium-high and bring to a low boil, then reduce heat to simmer and cook for 1½ to 2 hours. Drain and rinse.

Sauté onion in olive oil in a large stockpot on medium-high heat until translucent, about 5 minutes. Add remaining ingredients, including 2 cups of the bean cooking liquid (can be replaced with broth or water); cover and cook on medium heat, simmering, for 1 hour, stirring occasionally and adding bean cooking liquid, broth, or water as needed. Continue to simmer on low heat until ready to serve. Spoon into serving bowls and top with shredded cheese if desired.

Jewel and Bean Bake
6 servings

This recipe was originally named "Yam and Bean Bake," but after a little research, I learned that sweet potatoes and yams are not at all the same thing. While many of us use the terms interchangeably, yams actually have a wood-like, inedible outer peel, grow to up to 8 feet and 150 pounds, and are mostly grown in Africa. The sweet potatoes available in several varieties, with flesh ranging from yellow to orange, are what most of us are familiar with. So "Yam and Bean Bake" is now "Jewel and Bean Bake," in which the combination of luscious sweet potatoes, nutty black beans, and savory roasted poblano peppers results in a dish to meant to savor.

If you're not familiar with poblano peppers, they're a smallish, dark green variety popular in Mexican cooking. They're not too spicy when the seeds and stem are removed, but any pepper of your preference can be substituted if poblanos aren't available.

Ingredients:
- 2 Jewel sweet potatoes, peeled and chopped into potato salad–sized cubes (about 4 cups)
- 2 poblano peppers, stem and seeds removed, coarsely chopped
- Juice from 1 orange (approximately ¼ cup)
- 1 tablespoon coconut oil
- 1 tablespoon Bragg Liquid Aminos or soy sauce
- 2 tablespoons rice vinegar
- 1 teaspoon salt
- 1 teaspoon powdered or granulated garlic; *or* 2 cloves garlic, crushed
- ½ cup scallions, chopped
- 2 cups black beans, precooked

To prepare beans from scratch, soak for at least 8 hours or overnight. Drain and rinse beans, then add to a large stockpot and fill with water to cover the beans by at least 6 inches. Turn heat to medium-high and bring to a low boil, then reduce heat to simmer and cook for 1½ to 2 hours. Drain and rinse.

Preheat oven to 385°. Combine all ingredients except scallions and beans in a glass or metal roasting pan and cook, covered, for 30 to 40 minutes. Give it a stir once or twice to keep moistened. When cooked through, turn off the oven, add scallions and beans, and let sit for 15 minutes, uncovered. Remove from the oven and serve hot or warm.

Polenta Fiesta Layer Cake
6 to 8 servings

Made from ground corn, polenta is an Italian cooking staple; it cooks like a porridge, but then firms up to the point where it's sliceable. Layered with Southwest-style ingredients in this yummy casserole, it makes a delicious one-dish meal.

Ingredients:
- 2 cups organic corn polenta (often available in bulk at grocery stores)
- 6 to 6¼ cups water
- 2 cups black beans, precooked
- 1 avocado, chopped
- 1½ cups salsa (jarred is fine; choose your preference, from mild to hot)
- ½ cup Nada Cheese Topping (see page 146) or shredded Parmesan cheese
- 1 cup prepared guacamole for topping (optional)

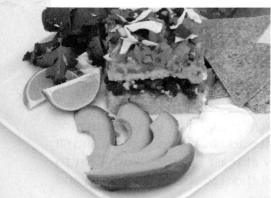

To prepare beans from scratch, soak for at least 8 hours or overnight. Drain and rinse beans, then add to a large stockpot and fill with water to cover the beans by at least 6 inches. Turn heat to medium-high and bring to a low boil, then reduce heat to simmer and cook for 1½ to 2 hours. Drain and rinse.

Prepare polenta according to instructions below. Polenta should be very thick but still stir-able. Add water, in very small increments, if needed. Spoon half of the cooked polenta mixture into the bottom of an ovenproof casserole dish. Mix together black beans and 1 cup of salsa. Gently spoon over the bottom layer of the polenta, and spread evenly. Add the rest of the polenta to cover the bean mixture, creating the top layer of the cake, and smooth it out so it's even.

Preheat your oven to 350°. Pop the casserole dish in and bake for 20 minutes uncovered. Remove from the oven and cool for 15 to 20 minutes. Top with remaining salsa, your choice of cheese topping, and serve.

Basic polenta preparation

Bring 6 cups water to a boil. Add 1 teaspoon salt and slowly pour in the 2 cups of polenta, stirring constantly with a fork to prevent lumps. Reduce heat to a gentle simmer, stirring for an additional 2 minutes.

Cover and cook for 40 to 45 minutes, stirring every 10 minutes.

Vegetarian Fajitas
4 servings

Similar to burritos, fajitas are fun to serve unassembled, with everyone customizing their own. A popular, flavorful party dish, serve it with brown rice to round out the meal.

Ingredients:
- 1 tablespoon olive or coconut oil
- 1 onion, coarsely chopped
- 1 medium pepper (red or green), coarsely chopped
- 1 teaspoon salt
- 1 teaspoon lime juice (fresh if available)
- 1 cup black beans, precooked
- 1 cup vegan or dairy cheese, shredded
- 1 cup of your favorite prepared salsa (or make your own; see page 134)
- 4 whole-wheat or other whole-grain tortillas

To prepare beans from scratch, soak for at least 8 hours or overnight. Drain and rinse beans, then add to a large stockpot and fill with water to cover the beans by at least 6 inches. Turn heat to medium-high and bring to a low boil, then reduce heat to simmer and cook for 1½ to 2 hours. Drain and rinse.

Sauté the peppers and onions in oil, salt, and lime juice for 5 to 8 minutes until onions are translucent, then transfer the mixture to a serving dish. Pour the beans right into the sauté pan (no need to rinse it), and add ¼ cup of salsa to the beans. Place back on medium heat and quickly warm up before transferring to a serving dish.

Warm your tortillas by wrapping them in a stack in aluminum foil and place in a preheated 350° oven until heated through, 15 to 20 minutes.

Serve your vegetable mixture, black beans, remaining salsa, cheese, and tortillas each in separate serving dishes. Layer the ingredients into your tortillas, roll, and enjoy!

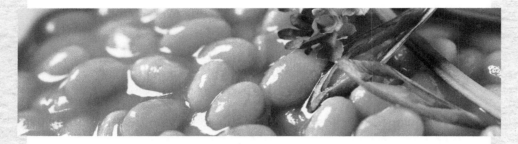

On the Side

If you've got some leftover beans and grains, there are lots of creative ways to use them. You can transform them into a whole new entree or whip up a yummy side dish. Either way, here are some simple recipes to get you going. As always, feel free to improvise with whatever you have on hand.

Parsnip Adzuki Fried Rice
4 servings

Looking for a delicious solution to leftover brown rice? Here it is! This easy dish is likely to be a favorite with the younger set, so think volume. The recipe is so simple that it lends itself to all kinds of tasty variations. And if you're not familiar with the nutty flavor of fresh parsnips—they look like white carrots—you're in for a pleasant surprise.

Ingredients:
- 1 tablespoon coconut oil
- 2 cups brown rice
- 1½ cups adzuki or black beans, precooked
- 1 parsnip, diced (about ½ cup)
- 1 cup cabbage, chopped
- 1 apple, cored and chopped (peeling is optional)
- 1 tablespoon Bragg Liquid Aminos
- ¼ teaspoon powdered or granulated garlic; *or* 1 clove garlic, crushed (optional)

- 1 teaspoon dried parsley or 3 teaspoons fresh parsley, chopped (optional; a blender or mini food processor makes the prep work easy)
- Salt to taste

Note: See the Bean Soaking and Cooking Chart on page 116 for bean preparation instructions.

In a large saucepan, sauté parsnip and cabbage in coconut oil for 5 minutes on medium heat, then add chopped apple and cook for 3 minutes more. Add rice, beans, Bragg Liquid Aminos, and seasonings; sauté for 2 minutes longer or until all ingredients are hot. Serve warm or hot.

Caribbean Black Beans
10 servings

As easy as they are versatile, these tasty beans make a great side dish, yummy burrito filling, or perfect complement to simple brown rice. Don't let the quantity scare you—you'll enjoy the leftovers all week!

Ingredients:
- 4 cups black beans, precooked
- 1 tablespoon coconut oil
- 1 mango, diced, or 1 cup frozen, chopped (optional)
- 1 teaspoon salt
- ¼ cup salsa (mango, papaya, or traditional; jarred or see page 134 to make your own)

To prepare beans from scratch, soak for at least 8 hours or overnight. Drain and rinse beans, then add to a large stockpot and fill with water to cover the beans by at least 6 inches. Turn heat to medium-high and bring to a low boil, then reduce heat to simmer and cook for 1½ to 2 hours. Drain and rinse.

In a medium-sized saucepan, heat coconut oil on medium. Add beans, and heat to desired temperature before mixing in remaining ingredients. Serve hot or cold.

Curried Brown Rice
4 servings

There's something so comforting about this lovely blend of rice, dried fruit, and nuts. Whether it's the unique trio of tastes or combination of textures, the results are delicious, and the curry seasoning gives an exotic flair. Add some teriyaki tofu and serve with a side of steamed or sautéed winter greens for a super-healthy meal.

Ingredients:
- 2 cups water
- 1 cup short-grain brown rice
- 2 tablespoons coconut or olive oil
- ½ cup red pepper, diced
- ½ cup white onion or scallions, chopped
- ½ cup frozen green peas
- ½ cup unsalted cashews, chopped (raw or roasted is fine)
- ½ cup raisins or dried cranberries
- 1 tablespoon Bragg Liquid Aminos
- 1½ teaspoons Curry Spice Blend (see page 144)
- ½ to 1 teaspoon salt

Prepare rice by bringing 2 cups of water to a low boil in a large saucepan. Add rice and return to a boil before reducing heat to low and covering the pan. Simmer for 40 minutes, add peppers and onions, then cover and cook for 5 minutes longer or until all water is absorbed. Remove from heat, add remaining ingredients, and serve.

Savory Baked Beans
8 to 10 servings

This rich, hearty dish is likely to be a family favorite. Perfect for chilly weather, it will warm your kitchen and make it smell good, then go on to warm your belly, too. The cooking time is substantial on this one, but once your beans are cooked á la stovetop, the rest of the prep work is a breeze. I like to whip up these vegetarian baked beans in large batches to make the most of the oven cooking time. They keep well refrigerated (up to 4 days) and freeze nicely for up to 2 months.

Ingredients:
- 6 cups kidney beans, precooked
- 1 cup tomato sauce (I like jarred tomatoes, but BPA-free canned is fine, too)
- 3 tablespoons organic ketchup
- ¼ cup molasses
- 1 teaspoon mustard (any kind)
- 1 teaspoon salt
- 1 teaspoon powdered or granulated garlic
- ¼ cup water, then additional as needed

To prepare beans from scratch, soak for at least 8 hours or overnight. Drain and rinse beans, then add to a large stockpot and fill with water to cover the beans by at least 6 inches. Turn heat to medium-high and bring to a low boil, then reduce heat to simmer and cook for 1½ hours. Drain and rinse.

Preheat oven to 385°. Combine all ingredients in glass casserole dish and cover. Bake for 2 to 3 hours, stirring once or twice during baking. Longer cooking means softer beans, but you may need to add water to keep a thick, but still-liquid consistency (think ketchup). Bake for the last 30 minutes with cover off, stirring once or twice.

Meatless Refried Beans
8 to 10 servings

This dish is so easy to prepare, and so versatile, too. And you may well find it's a kid-friendly favorite! Serve alongside brown rice and top with dairy-free cheese for an updated version of a classic combination that's flat-out delicious.

Ingredients:
- 6 cups kidney or pinto beans, precooked until soft
- 2 to 3 tablespoons coconut oil

- 3 teaspoons chili powder
- 2 teaspoons salt
- ½ cup water as needed

To prepare beans from scratch, soak for at least 8 hours or overnight. Drain and rinse beans, then add to a large stockpot and fill with water to cover the beans by at least 6 inches. Turn heat to medium-high and bring to a low boil, then reduce heat to simmer and cook for 1½ hours.

Heat coconut oil in a large skillet over medium heat. Add beans and ¼ cup water, then mash beans in the pan with a potato masher to desired consistency (it's fine to leave some whole). Add remaining ingredients and sauté for 5 to 10 minutes, adding remaining ¼ cup water as needed. Beans should be soft but not soupy.

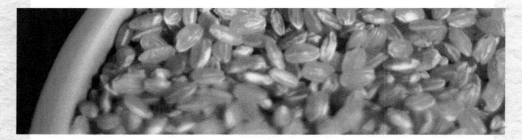

Grains

Nothing completes a bean-and-greens meal like healthy whole grains. Together beans and grains form a complete high-quality protein chain. Brown rice is always a great standby, but if you find yourself in need of some culinary inspiration, then this section is just the place to get it. Much as I love my brown rice, there are many wonderful alternatives which are just as wholesome, inexpensive, and easy to prepare.

Quinoa (pronounced "keen-wah") is fast becoming a go-to staple among the home-cooking set. New to the wonders of quinoa? Similar to couscous in size and texture, quinoa is actually a relative of leafy green vegetables like spinach and Swiss chard. Since it's loaded with protein and other nutrients, it can be a healthier alternative to your everyday side dish. It's super-tasty *and* as easy to prepare as a pot of rice, with which it can usually be used interchangeably.

Black rice, so named for its signature color and also known as purple rice or forbidden rice, is another rising star. This delicious sticky-rice variety is increasingly finding its way to menus and bulk bins. High in nutrients (including potent anti-inflammatory properties) and wonderfully flavorful, it's just as simple to make as brown or white rice, and adds an exotic twist to any meal.

For all the great flavor and even more health benefits, try barley as another rice alternative. Barley is the highest-fiber whole grain, with even more cholesterol-reducing properties than oats. It's prepared similarly to brown rice, but the heartier texture makes a nice base for soups, stews, or even the occasional salad.

You may want to continue along your great grain discovery mission with adventurous options like farro, kamut, or any of the other exciting grain alternatives that are finally making their way into the mainstream. With all these options, it's easy to be creative, so have fun!

Basic Brown Rice
4 servings

This is such a staple in our house. It's no more complicated to make than dried pasta, but when I saw brown rice sold precooked and frozen, I realized it's possible that not everyone has discovered this. Leftover rice is easy to rejuvenate by steaming, covered, in a couple of tablespoons of water. Double or triple this recipe as needed.

Ingredients:
- 1 cup brown rice (short- or medium-grain are good choices)
- 2¼ cups water
- 1 teaspoon salt
- 1 tablespoon olive, coconut, or sesame oil (optional)
- 1 tablespoon Bragg Liquid Aminos or tamari sauce (optional)

Bring water to a boil in a medium-sized saucepan. Add rice and return just briefly to simmer. Cover and reduce heat. Cook for 45 to 50 minutes until water is absorbed. Let sit covered for 5 to 10 minutes longer, then remove from heat and stir in remaining ingredients. Serve warm or hot.

Quinoa Garsnippity
6 servings

This scrumptious and satisfying dish features garnet sweet potatoes and parsnips—hence the jazzy name!

Quinoa salads like this one are easy to make by adding your vegetables to the quinoa right before it's done cooking; toss in your seasonings at the end and you're done in one dish. This recipe is hearty enough to serve as an entree, but it's also great as a side dish. For a yummy and versatile lunch base, top it with greens and you're good to go.

Ingredients:
- 2 cups quinoa, soaked for at least 4 hours before cooking
- ½ large sweet potato or 2 carrots (unpeeled is fine), diced into small cubes
- 1 medium parsnip, diced into small cubes
- 1 cup mung beans, precooked (soaking up to 24 hours is optional)
- ¼ cup cilantro, finely chopped (a spice grinder or mini food processor is great for this)
- 2 tablespoons Bragg Liquid Aminos
- 1 tablespoon sesame oil
- ½ to 1 teaspoon salt to taste
- 1 tablespoon sweet chili sauce (available in most health-food or Asian specialty stores)

Drain and rinse beans, then add to a large stockpot and fill with water to cover the beans by at least 6 inches. Turn heat to medium-high and bring to a low boil, then reduce heat to simmer and cook for 20 to 30 minutes if soaked, or 45 to 60 minutes if not. Drain and rinse.

Drain and rinse quinoa after soaking. Place with 2 cups of water into a large saucepan and bring to a simmer. Cook for 10 minutes, adding ¼ cup more water if all liquid is absorbed, then add chopped parsnip, sweet potato or carrot, and cilantro, and cook for 5 minutes more. Add remaining ingredients and serve hot or cold.

Forbidden Rice Ginger Salad
6 servings

The chewy texture of forbidden, or black, rice gives this dish a heartier feel, and tempered with the mellow flavor of sweet potatoes, it's fabulous served hot or cold. And it's just as delicious the next day or so.

Ingredients:
Salad:
- 1½ cups forbidden/black rice
- 3 cups water
- 6 scallions, finely chopped (approximately ¾ cup)
- 1 sweet potato, cut into small cubes
- 1 teaspoon salt

Dressing:
- ¼ cup freshly squeezed orange juice
- 1 to 2 tablespoons fresh ginger, finely grated, or 2 teaspoons powdered ginger
- 1 tablespoon sesame oil
- 2 tablespoons rice vinegar
- 1 tablespoon honey
- 1 teaspoon salt

Bring water to a boil and add the rice. Immediately reduce heat to low and cover. Cook for 10 minutes, then add sweet potato and cook for 10 to 15 minutes longer or until potato is tender and rice is chewy. Mix in the scallions and remove from heat. Add dressing ingredients to a blender or food processor and puree for a few minutes until smooth. Pour over salad and serve.

Barley Pilaf
6 servings

A flavorful twist on a culinary classic. Serve as a hearty side dish alongside a basic veggie stir-fry for a colorful, flavorful meal.

Ingredients:
- 1 tablespoon walnut or olive oil
- 1 onion, chopped (approximately 1 cup)
- 1 carrot, diced
- 1¾ cup pearled barley
- 3 cups water
- 2 cubes or tablespoons vegetable bouillon
- 2 tablespoons rice vinegar
- 1 clove garlic, crushed; *or* 1 teaspoon powdered or granulated garlic
- 1 teaspoon salt or to taste
- Freshly ground pepper, to taste
- 1 cup green peas, fresh or frozen
- ½ cup slivered, unsalted almonds

Add the oil to a large sauté pan on medium heat. Add onion, barley, and carrot and sauté the mixture, stirring frequently, until the barley is golden, about 5 minutes. Add the water, bouillon, vinegar, and seasonings. Cover and cook until the barley is tender, about 60 to 75 minutes. Add the peas and almonds, then let cool slightly before serving.

Veggie Fried Rice
4 servings

This is my favorite dish to make with leftover rice, and I cook extra just to make sure I have enough to prepare it the next day. My kids adore this yummy rice—so to avoid potential squabbles over seconds, I'm careful to make more than enough to go around.

Ingredients:
- 2 cups cooked brown rice
- 2 tablespoons coconut oil
- 1 egg, cracked into a bowl and whisked with 1 teaspoon water (optional)
- ¼ cup onion, leek, or chives, chopped
- ½ cup celery, finely chopped
- ½ cup cabbage, finely chopped (optional)
- 3 tablespoons Savory Sauce Blend (see page 141); *or* 1 tablespoon Bragg Liquid Aminos, 1 tablespoon rice vinegar, and 2 teaspoons Asian fish sauce
- ½ teaspoon salt
- 1 teaspoon powdered or granulated garlic (optional)

Note: To prepare Basic Brown Rice, visit page 189.

Heat 1 tablespoon coconut oil in a large sauté pan over medium-high heat. Add egg, if using, and quickly fry until cooked through. Remove from pan and put aside. Scrape any remaining food from the pan, add remaining oil, and return to medium heat. Add chopped vegetables and stir in Savory Sauce Blend. Cook until tender, 5 to 7 minutes. Add rice and remaining ingredients and sauté until heated through, 2 to 4 minutes. Remove from heat and serve right away.

Springtime Quinoa
4 to 6 servings

Light, easy, and super-healthy, this side salad dish can also take center stage as a main course when served over mixed greens. Or try filling a bowl halfway full of Springtime Quinoa, then top with some hot tomato soup for a warm and nourishing evening meal.

Ingredients:
- 1 cup quinoa (any variety will do)
- 2 cups water
- 1 small red onion (skin removed) or 1 large leek bulb, coarsely chopped
- 1 fennel bulb, coarsely chopped

- 1 small red or green pepper, seeded and chopped
- 3 to 5 tablespoons of your choice of Ginger Peanut Sauce (see page 202), Cilantro Mint Sauce (see page 138), or Basil Pesto Sauce (see page 144)

Bring water to boiling in a medium saucepan, add quinoa, and return to simmering. Reduce heat to low, cover, and cook for 15 to 20 minutes or until most of the water is absorbed. Toss in onion, fennel, and pepper; cover and cook at lowest possible temperature for 5 more minutes, stirring halfway through and adding more water if needed to prevent browning.

Remove from burner and add your choice of sauce, seasoned to taste. Serve warm or at room temperature.

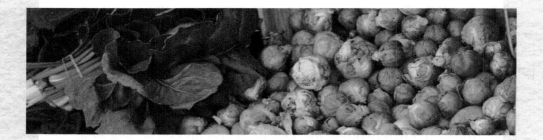

Vegetables

For many, vegetables are kind of an afterthought, typically the second act to a meaty main event. If this sounds like you, and you're looking to rethink your relationship with garden fare, I've included some easy, favorite veggie recipes designed to surprise you. And if you're used to seasoning with nothing but salt, a squeeze of lemon, and maybe a splash of soy sauce or Bragg's, you'll be delighted at how satisfying a little culinary novelty can be.

Butternut Squash with Tahini
8 servings

Fresh squash can look intimidating to the uninitiated, but there's really nothing to worry about; it can be super-easy to prepare. Cutting it up is usually the hardest part of the project. Using a sharp, sturdy knife, slice your squash lengthwise, scrape out the seeds with a spoon (use a serrated one if you have it), and you're ready to go.

In this dish, the taste combination is fabulous. Serve it with a garlicky sautéed green and your favorite grain for a hearty and wholesome meal.

Ingredients:
- 1- to 2-pound butternut squash, sliced lengthwise, seeds removed
- ¼ cup tahini
- 2 teaspoons salt
- 2 teaspoons powdered or granulated garlic

Heat oven to 375°. Place both halves of squash, cut side down, on a cookie or baking sheet (rimmed is optional) and bake for 45 minutes, until skin is browned and inside is very soft. Remove from heat and cool for 15 minutes before scooping the flesh out of the shell and into a large serving bowl. Add remaining ingredients, stirring until smooth and creamy in texture, then serve.

Orange Ginger Carrots
4 to 6 servings

Ingredients:
- 1 pound carrots (peeled optional), cut matchstick style
- ½ cup fresh-squeezed orange juice
- 2 tablespoons tamari or Bragg Liquid Aminos
- 1 teaspoon fresh ginger, grated
- 2 tablespoons honey
- ½ teaspoon salt (optional or to taste)

Steam carrots in 1 inch of water in large saucepan for 5 minutes. Drain water and add remaining ingredients. Bring to a simmer over medium heat and cook uncovered, stirring often, until the liquid is reduced to about 1 tablespoon. Serve hot or cold.

Garlicky Greens
4 servings

Ever feel intimidated by the big bunches of kale, chard, or collards you see at the market? Don't be! They're so easy to cook, and the nutritional punch is too good to ignore. An easy trick for de-stemming your hearty greens is to hold the main stalk in one hand and strip the leaf from the stem all the way up with the other hand.

Ingredients:
- 1 head of kale, Swiss chard, or collard greens, stems removed and torn into bite-sized pieces
- 2 tablespoons olive oil
- ½ teaspoon salt
- 4 cloves garlic, crushed; *or* 2 teaspoons powdered or granulated garlic
- 2 tablespoons balsamic vinegar or 1 tablespoon lemon juice (fresh if available)
- 3 tablespoons slivered almonds (optional)

Place olive oil in a large sauté pan over medium-high heat. Add greens and salt, and sauté, stirring continuously until color gets bright and they begin to wilt, about 5 minutes. Add garlic and cook for 2 to 3 minutes more until garlic begins to brown, adding tablespoons of water as needed to avoid burning if mixture gets dry. Add balsamic vinegar or lemon juice and remove from heat. Serve right away.

Asian-style Green Beans
4 to 6 servings

These are a classic kids' favorite. Beans can be cooked lightly or lots, depending on preference. Quick green bean prep tip: there's no need for fancy trimming; simply pinch the stem end off but leave the tender tip on the other end.

Ingredients:
- 1 pound fresh green beans, stems removed
- 2 scallions, diced
- 2 to 3 teaspoons fresh ginger, minced or grated
- 1 clove garlic, crushed; *or* 1 teaspoon powdered or granulated garlic
- 3 tablespoons Savory Sauce Blend (see page 141); *or* 1 tablespoon each Bragg Liquid Aminos and rice vinegar, plus 1 teaspoon Asian fish sauce (optional)
- 1 teaspoon sesame oil (optional)

Place ½ inch of water in large sauté pan and bring to a simmer. Add beans and cook for 3 to 5 minutes. Drain and return to the stovetop. Add remaining ingredients and stir-fry for 3 to 5 minutes longer. When cooked to preferred level of tenderness, remove and serve immediately.

Roasted Curried Cauliflower
4 servings

Simple and delicious. Oven roasting is an easy way to prepare this savory side dish.

Ingredients:
- 1 small head cauliflower, cored and cut into large florets
- 2 tablespoons olive oil
- 2 teaspoons Curry Spice Blend (see page 144)
- 1 teaspoon salt

Preheat oven to 385°. Toss all ingredients in a bowl and spread in a single layer onto a rimmed baking sheet. Cook for about 30 minutes or until cauliflower is tender and lightly browned. Serve immediately.

Lemony Broccoli
4 servings

Broccoli is my go-to veggie. It's available everywhere, usually pretty fresh due to its high popularity, and easy to prepare. Here's a good, basic, delicious recipe.

Ingredients:
- 1 head broccoli, stem removed, the rest separated into large florets
- 2 cloves garlic, crushed; *or* 1 teaspoon powdered or granulated garlic
- 2 tablespoons olive oil
- 2 tablespoons Bragg Liquid Aminos
- 1 tablespoon lemon juice (fresh if available)
- 1 teaspoon salt

Place ½ inch of water into a saucepan and bring to a simmer over medium heat. Add broccoli and steam for 5 minutes. Drain liquid and add remaining ingredients. Return to heat and sauté for 2 to 5 minutes longer. Serve hot or at room temperature.

Nutty Brussels Sprout Curry Sauté
6 servings

Brussels sprouts have gotten a bad rap over the years, largely due to improper handling. When cooked al dente and nicely seasoned, even my kids appreciate these super-nutritious crucifers. So push aside any preconceptions, try this simple sauté, and decide for yourself!

Ingredients:
- 1 pound Brussels sprouts, woody stems trimmed off, halved
- 2 tablespoons olive oil
- 3 tablespoons Savory Sauce Blend (see page 141); *or* 1 tablespoon each Bragg Liquid Aminos and rice vinegar, plus 1 teaspoon Asian fish sauce (optional)
- ¼ cup walnuts
- ½ teaspoon powdered or granulated garlic
- 1 tablespoon lemon juice (fresh if available)
- ½ teaspoon lemon zest (optional)

Add ½ inch of water to a sauté or saucepan and bring to a simmer. Add Brussels sprouts and steam, covered, for 10 to 15 minutes until cooked through. Drain water, add oil, and return to heat. Add remaining ingredients and stir-fry for 5 minutes. Remove from heat and serve.

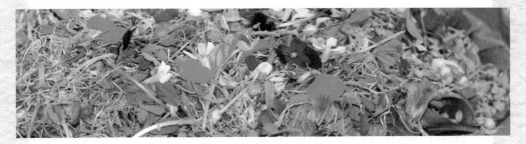

Sprouts

The age-old practice of sprouting seeds and legumes for the additional health benefits they're known to offer was—until recently—nearly forgotten. But new research on the important nutritional benefits of microgreens, along with the growing trend toward urban gardening, has, to my delight, reinvigorated this lost art. Feel free to refer back to Chapter 17 for detailed instructions on easy kitchen sprouting. You'll be amazed at both the simplicity of the process, and the scrumptious (and economical) results.

Sprouted Wheat Breakfast Cookies
20 to 30 small cookies

Sprouted wheat is the real deal, retaining all the nutrients of the entire wheat berry without any of the added fillers and preservatives. Sprouting breaks down the starches in grains into simple sugars so that your body can digest them more easily, including that notoriously difficult-to-digest wheat protein, gluten. These cookies are easily transportable, wonderfully tasty, highly nutritious, and sugar-free. A perfect breakfast treat!

Ingredients:
- 2 cups sprouted soft-wheat berries
- ½ teaspoon salt
- 1 teaspoon cinnamon
- 1 teaspoon stevia powder
- 1 teaspoon vanilla extract
- 1 cup coconut, shredded
- 1 cup raisins or dried cranberries
- 1 cup nuts (walnuts or pecans), chopped

Preheat oven to 250°. Add sprouted wheat berries, salt, stevia, cinnamon, and vanilla to a blender (you'll need a heavy-duty one for this job) or food processor and pulverize until smooth. Transfer to a large bowl, and knead in the remaining ingredients until fully incorporated.

Grease a cookie sheet with coconut oil. Keeping your hands moist to prevent sticking, shape cookie dough into 1-inch balls, then flatten into little disks. Bake for 1½ to 2 hours until firm, but still moist. Store cookies in a glass jar for up to 1 week, or in the freezer for up to 3 months.

Kale, Sweet Potato, and Sprout Salad with Miso Dressing

6 to 8 servings

Minimalist that I am, I wasn't remotely interested in cooking with steamer baskets until I learned this incredible recipe in a cooking class. I love that the steamer method is low-tech, easy to learn, and *fast.* At home I use a bamboo steamer, which creates an interesting and not unpleasant scent while steaming.

You'll need two stackable steamer baskets for this dish.

Ingredients:
- 2 heads of kale, Swiss chard, or collard greens, stemmed and chopped
- 1 large garnet sweet potato, cut into quarters lengthwise and then into ½-inch slices
- ½ cup scallions, chopped
- 2 cups mung bean sprouts
- ¼ to ½ cup Ginger Miso Dressing (see page 143)

Add 6 inches of water to a large saucepan and bring it to a boil. Place the sweet potato slices on the bottom steamer basket, and greens on the other one. Place the sweet potato basket over the pot of water and cover; steam for 7 minutes. Add the greens layer, cover, and steam for 5 minutes longer. Check the sweet potato slices for doneness, and once tender, remove from heat.

Add to a bowl, toss in the scallions, and let cool for 20 minutes or longer before tossing in sprouts and adding dressing. Serve salad at room temperature or make ahead and refrigerate, adding dressing right before serving.

Mung Bean Crunch
4 to 6 servings

This fresh, zesty salad is a great way to get started with sprouts. Mung beans are simple to sprout, requiring only a few days before they're ready to use. They're incredibly nutritious and surprisingly tasty, too.

Ingredients:
- 3 to 4 cups mung bean sprouts
- ½ cup scallions, chopped
- 1 cup green cabbage, shredded
- ½ teaspoon salt
- ¼ cup Cilantro Mint Sauce (see page 138)
- ½ cup sliced almonds or chopped peanuts
- 1 tablespoon Asian fish sauce (optional)
- 1 tablespoon Bragg Liquid Aminos
- 1 teaspoon chili sauce (optional)
- 1 cup chopped tofu (optional)

In a large salad bowl, combine all ingredients and mix well. Let stand for 20 minutes or so before serving.

Fresh Thai Spring Rolls with Ginger Peanut Sauce
8 servings

I'll admit, I'm a spring-roll junkie—I love the flavor and texture combinations, and when prepared with tofu and peanuts, they make a wonderfully light and satisfying meal. As with so many of the Beanalicious recipes, you can get creative with the ingredients here, too. Luckily, those mysterious rice wrappers are easier to prepare then you might imagine: just soak to soften, then wrap away!

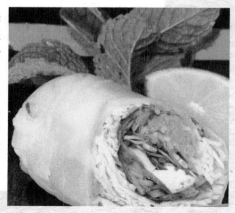

Ingredients:
- 8 rice wrappers (available in the Asian-foods section of most grocery stores)
- 2 cups alfalfa or radish sprouts
- 2 cups green-leaf lettuce leaves; *or* green cabbage, finely shredded
- 2 large carrots, shredded
- 3 tablespoons fresh mint leaves, chopped (a blender or mini food processor is great for this)
- 3 tablespoons fresh cilantro, chopped (see above)
- 3 tablespoons unsalted peanuts, raw or roasted, chopped
- 6 ounces firm tofu, plain or teriyaki-flavored, cut into 16 thin strips
- 1 avocado, seed and peel removed, cut into 16 thin strips (optional)
- Ginger Peanut Sauce for dipping (see page 202)

Fill a large bowl with warm water. Dip a wrapper into the warm water for just a second or two to soften, then lay it flat and get ready to wrap. In a row across the center, place 2 tofu strips, an avocado strip, ¼ cup sprouts, a lettuce leaf or ¼ cup cabbage, ¼ cup carrots; then sprinkle with mint and cilantro, leaving about 2 inches on either side of the wrap without any ingredients. Fold the "naked" sides inward, then tightly roll the wrapper. Repeat with remaining ingredients. Serve with Ginger Peanut Sauce.

Agape Salad
8 servings

Spouting brings out the best in your lentils. Sprouted lentils are not only easier to digest, they're nutty, nourishing, and delicious. The sprouting increases digestibility (so you can hold the Beano), produces vitamin C, *and* increases vitamin B and carotene content.

This satisfying salad is a healthy, nutritious entree or side dish. Kale and cabbage are interchangeable here, depending on taste and availability. Pair it with brown rice and a roasted butternut squash for a fabulous meal.

Ingredients:
- 3 cups raw, sprouted lentils or 2 cups dried green lentils
- 1½ cup dinosaur kale or cabbage, chopped
- ½ cup mild red or white onion, diced
- ½ to 1 whole avocado, chopped (optional)
- ½ cup organic smoked tofu, chopped (use extra-firm unflavored if smoked is unavailable)
- 1 cup sunflower seeds or walnuts

Dressing:
- ¼ cup Savory Sauce Blend (see page 141); or 3 tablespoons each Bragg Liquid Aminos and rice vinegar and 2 teaspoons Asian fish sauce
- 3 tablespoons olive oil
- ½ to 1 teaspoon powdered or granulated garlic

Prepare raw lentils by steaming in ½ inch of water for 4 to 8 minutes, depending on how soft you like them, or cook dried lentils according to the Bean Soaking and Cooking Chart on page 116.

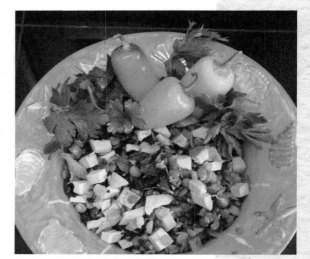

Drain cooked lentils and leave them in the pot on the stove. Mix in onion and kale or cabbage; immediately cover for 5 minutes. Prepare dressing in a large bowl and toss in lentil mixture. Add tofu and toss. Gently toss in avocado (if using); when cool, top with sunflower seeds or walnuts and serve.

Spicy Sprout Salad
6 to 8 servings

A salad worth sprouting for! Use sprouted mung or adzuki beans for an appealing twist on the traditional chopped-veggie salad, this time with all the amazing health benefits of sprouts.

Ingredients:
- 4 cups sprouted adzuki or mung beans
- 2 large fennel bulbs, thinly sliced and chopped to the same length as sprouts
- ½ cup scallions, thinly sliced
- ¼ cup cilantro, chopped (a coffee grinder or mini food processor is good for this)
- ½ to ¾ cup Ginger Miso Dressing (see page 143)

Combine all ingredients and serve.

Red Lentil Kitcharee
6 to 8 servings

Kitcharee is the Hindi word for "mess" or "mixture," and this classic Indian dish is a really wholesome blend of fiber, healthy fats, and healing spices, perfect for when you need some extra energy or nourishment. Mine is a pared-down version: to save some steps, I've substituted coconut oil for the traditionally used ghee (refined butter) and my Curry Spice Blend for the variety of spices typically used. The red lentils, often referred to as dal, cook quickly and help the mixture to thicken into a hearty, fragrant, almost porridge-style stew. Delicious!

Ingredients:
- ¾ cup red lentils
- 1½ cups short-grain brown basmati rice
- 2 tablespoons coconut oil
- 3 to 4 teaspoons Curry Spice Blend (see page 144)
- 1 teaspoon salt

- 1 cube or 1 teaspoon vegetable bouillon
- 6 to 8 cups water
- 3 to 4 cups diced vegetables, such as carrots, zucchini, and/or cauliflower
- 2 cups mung bean sprouts

Add lentils and rice to a colander and rinse well until water runs clear. Add coconut oil to a large pot and warm to melt. Add the Curry Spice Blend, rice, and lentils; stir to heat through and add 6 cups of water. Bring to a simmer over medium heat, cover, and cook for about 1 hour, or until the beans and rice are soft. Add salt, bouillon, and diced vegetables and cook 15 minutes more, adding more water as needed if you prefer a soupier consistency. Stir in the bean sprouts in the last 3 to 5 minutes before removing from the stove. Serve warm.

Sprouted Adzuki Mushroom Medley
4 to 6 servings

Sprouted legumes become so tender you can eat them raw or lightly steamed, which removes any hint of starchiness. Sprouting enhances flavor and helps with digestion, so it's a great way to get the most from your beans. This simple stir-fry incorporates fresh mushrooms in a delectable combination of flavors perfectly complemented by a side of brown rice.

Ingredients:
- 3 cups sprouted adzuki or mung beans
- 1 tablespoon coconut or olive oil
- ½ cup celery, chopped
- ½ cup onion, any variety, coarsely chopped
- 1 cup shitake mushrooms (if unavailable, use brown mushrooms), sliced
- ¼ cup Basil Pesto (see page 144)

Add ½ inch of water to a large sauté pan and bring to a simmer. Add adzuki or mung beans and steam 5 minutes, then drain. Add oil to the same pan and reheat before adding celery, onions, and mushrooms; sauté for 5 to 8 minutes longer, until veggies are tender. Toss in pesto and serve.

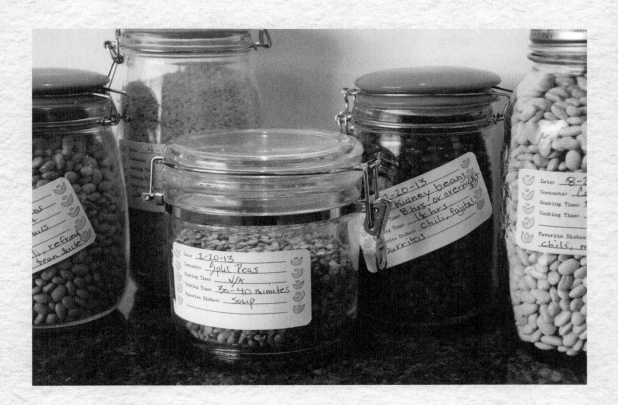

Resources and Information for Beanalicious Living

Books

Information and advocacy

Diet for a Small Planet by Frances Moore Lappé

EcoMind: Changing the Way We Think, to Create the World We Want by Frances Moore Lappé

The Food Revolution: How Your Diet Can Help Save Your Life and Our World by John Robbins

Diet for a New America: How Your Food Choices Affect Your Health, Happiness and the Future of Life on Earth by John Robbins

In Defense of Food: An Eater's Manifesto by Michael Pollan

The Omnivore's Dilemma: A Natural History of Four Meals by Michael Pollan

Fast Food Nation: The Dark Side of the All-American Meal by Eric Schlosser

The Unhealthy Truth: One Mother's Shocking Investigation into the Dangers of America's Food Supply—and What Every Family Can Do to Protect Itself by Robyn O'Brien and Rachel Kranz

Righteous Porkchop: Finding a Life and Good Food Beyond Factory Farms by Nicolette Hahn Niman

Appetite for Profit: How the Food Industry Undermines Our Health and How to Fight Back by Michele Simon

The Willpower Instinct: How Self-control Works, Why It Matters, and What You Can Do to Get More of It by Kelly McGonigal, Ph.D.

Healthy Living

The New Good Life: Living Better Than Ever in an Age of Less by John Robbins

Veganist: Lose Weight, Get Healthy, Change the World by Kathy Freston

Crazy Sexy Diet: Eat Your Veggies, Ignite Your Spark, and Live Like You Mean It! by Kris Carr

The Happiness Diet: A Nutritional Prescription for a Sharp Brain, Balanced Mood, and Lean, Energized Body by Tyler Graham and Drew Ramsey, M.D.

Living Room Revolution: A Handbook for Conversation, Community and the Common Good by Cecile Andrews

Prevent and Reverse Heart Disease: The Revolutionary, Scientifically Proven,

Nutrition-based Cure by Caldwell B. Esselstyn, Jr., M.D.

Body for Life: 12 Weeks to Mental and Physical Strength by Bill Phillips

Nutrition

Eat, Drink, and Be Healthy: The Harvard Medical School Guide to Healthy Eating by Walter C. Willett, M.D., and P.J. Skerrett

The China Study: The Most Comprehensive Study of Nutrition Ever Conducted and the Startling Implications for Diet, Weight Loss, and Long-term Health by T. Colin Campbell, Ph.D., and Thomas M. Campbell II

Forks Over Knives: The Plant-based Way to Health, edited by Gene Stone

Food Rules: An Eater's Manual by Michael Pollan

Superimmunity for Kids: What to Feed Your Children to Keep Them Healthy Now, and Prevent Disease in Their Future by Leo Galland, M.D., with Dian Dincin Buchman, Ph.D.

Thrive: The Vegan Nutrition Guide to Optimal Performance in Sports and Life by Brendan Brazier

The Complete Idiot's Guide to Plant-based Nutrition by Julieanna Hever, M.S., R.D., C.P.T.

What to Eat by Marion Nestle

Eat to Live: The Amazing Nutrient-rich Program for Fast and Sustained Weight Loss by Joel Furhman, M.D.

Dr. Dean Ornish's Program for Reversing Heart Disease: The Only System Scientifically Proven to Reverse Heart Disease Without Drugs or Surgery by Dean Ornish, M.D.

The Sprouting Book: How to Grow and Use Sprouts to Maximize Your Health and Vitality by Ann Wigmore

The Encyclopedia of Healing Foods by Michael Murray, N.D., and Joseph Pizzorno, N.D., with Lara Pizzorno, M.A., L.M.T.

Breaking Free from Emotional Eating by Geneen Roth

101 Foods That Could Save Your Life by David Grotto, R.D., L.D.N.

Cookbooks

How to Cook Everything Vegetarian: Simple Meatless Recipes for Great Food by Mark Bittman

Food Matters: A Guide to Conscious Eating with More Than 75 Recipes by Mark Bittman

Moosewood Cookbook by Molly Katzen

The Sprouted Kitchen: A Tastier Take on Whole Foods by Sara Forte

Bean by Bean: A Cookbook by Crescent Dragonwagon

Forks Over Knives: The Cookbook: Over 300 Recipes for Plant-based Eating All Through the Year by Del Sroufe

Sproutman's Kitchen Garden Cookbook by Steve Meyerowitz

Milks Alive: 140 Delicious and Nutritious Recipes for Fresh Nut and Seed Milks by Rita Rivera

The Ayurvedic Vegan Kitchen: Finding Harmony Through Food by Talya Lutzker

Cookbooks for Kids

Pretend Soup and Other Real Recipes: A Cookbook for Preschoolers and Up by Mollie Katzen and Ann. L. Henderson

Salad People and More Real Recipes: A New Cookbook for Preschoolers and Up by Mollie Katzen

Honest Pretzels: And 64 Other Amazing Recipes for Kids Who Love to Cook by Mollie Katzen

Once Upon a Recipe: Great Food for Kids of All Ages by Karen Green

Websites

Nutrition

Harvard School of Public Health

Healthy Eating Plate and Healthy Eating Pyramid

http://www.hsph.harvard.edu/nutritionsource/pyramid

Physicians Committee for Responsible Medicine, http://www.pcrm.org

Andrew Weil, M.D., http://www.drweil.com

Nutrition Action Health Letter, http://www.cspinet.org/nah

Jeff Novick, M.S., R.D., L.D., L.N., http://www.jeffnovick.com

Chef Jenny Brewer, http://www.nourishingnutrition.com

Weston A. Price Foundation, http://www.westonaprice.org

Information and advocacy

Meat Free Monday, http://meatfreemondays.com/

The Food Revolution Network. http://www.foodrevolution.org

Friends of the Earth, http://www.foe.org

Organic Consumers Association, http://www.organicconsumers.org

Environmental Working Group, http://www.ewg.org

Center for Food Safety, http://www.centerforfoodsafety.org

Local living (and eating)

LocalHarvest, http://www.localharvest.org

Transition United States, http://www.transitionus.org

Edible Communities Publications, http://www.ediblecommunities.com

Recipes

Savvy Vegetarian, http://www.savvyvegetarian.com

VegNews, http://www.vegnews.com

Whole Living, http://www.wholeliving.com

Products and Supplies

Green Sprout Kit, http://www.sustainablesantacruz.com

http://www.ElizabethBorelli.com

Mountain Rose Herbs, http://www.mountainroseherbs.com

Bragg Liquid Aminos, http://www.bragg.com

Organic India, http://www.organicindia.com

Mendocino Sea Vegetable Company, http://www.seaweed.net

HealthForce Nutritionals, http://healthforce.com

Acknowledgements

My path to the whole-foods lifestyle was not a linear one. Ten years ago, I thought that popping a multivitamin once a day covered any nutritional needs not met by low-cal frozen dinners. Yet my concern for the environment, combined with commitment to wellness education, brought to light troubling truths about foods we routinely consume with barely a second glance (beyond checking their fat and calorie count).

Inspired by the work of Frances Moore Lappé, John Robbins, and Marion Nestle, I gradually became aware that the path to environmental sustainability begins in the kitchen. Too, I realized that it's not just Big Oil causing the problem; factory farms are also one of the top industrial polluters. And since overly refined, processed foods are a key culprit in rising rates of diet-related diseases, I learned that it's best to avoid them. Yet in sharing this information with other equally time-constrained friends, it became clear to me that while lots of people recognize the problem, they feel trapped. They don't have time to cook from scratch, they don't even know how, and they buy "natural" foods anyway so they don't feel the problem is personally relevant.

All of which explains the genesis of this book. I wanted to succinctly and systematically provide factual information about deceptive practices in the marketing of both mainstream and "natural" foods; to offer easy, affordable alternatives; and most importantly, to provide efficient strategies and resources to help streamline the process.

Fortunately I didn't need to pave the path alone. Many great minds were referenced in the making of *Beanalicious Living* (as you can see in the Resource section), with experts such as Dr. Joel Fuhrman, Dr. Dean Ornish, and Dr. T. Colin Campbell foremost among them. I also owe a show of appreciation to the tremendous influence of authors Michael Pollan and Mark Bittman for helping to make complicated cooking passé, leaving plenty of room for simple basics like beans.

On a personal note, I'd like to thank amazing editors Lisa Pliscou and Karen Kibler for helping to shape my vision into words, publisher Nancy Cleary of Wyatt-MacKenzie Publishing for packaging it so beautifully, and consultant Lisa Orrell for showing me the best path for getting here. Thank you, Rebecca Stark, for lending your talented eye to the many photo shoots it took to pull this vision together, and to New Leaf Community Markets for sharing their beautiful kitchen for the *Beanalicious Living* cover image. A shout-out to Renae Stowell and Mary Pellegrino for assisting with much of the recipe test cooking, and to all the friends who sat through those evenings of course after course of bean dishes and never once asked, "Where's the beef?"

Thank you, too, to my progressive parents for raising their children (mostly) fast-food-free during the dawn of the TV-dinner era and for their support and encouragement through my adventures in authorship! And—last but not least—a giant thanks to my patient husband and open-minded children for their willingness to eat outside the box, even during my most experimental phases, You guys rock!

Index

About the Author

Elizabeth Borelli has extensive experience in natural wellness education and advocacy. Her earlier career in the high-tech world didn't prepare her for the plunge into parenting, which opened her eyes to more than just motherhood. Her family's health and wellness immediately jumped to priority #1. She was also inspired to do her part to take care of the planet, and in 2004 she founded the green-living online resource and retailer Nubius Organics, which paved the way for a journey of transformation which has spanned the past decade. The more she learned about green living, the more convinced Elizabeth became that the road to both personal and planetary health begins in the kitchen.

Elizabeth's website, www.ElizabethBorelli.com, fulfills her goal of sharing with readers news, ideas, and tips for a healthy lifestyle, and to help them make informed choices in fun and easy ways.

Her passion for educating people—and busy people in particular!—on the importance of healthy eating has prompted her to align with experts such as John Robbins, Frances Moore Lappé, Summer Rayne Oaks, and Simran Sethi, all of whom she has hosted at events in Santa Cruz, California, as part of her advocacy work. Elizabeth regularly contributes to online wellness-related forums, and her work has been featured on MindBodyGreen.com, My.CrazySexyLife.com, and Care2.com. She is a member of Transition Santa Cruz, an organization supporting the ongoing transition to a vibrant, locally based economy, and also serves on the Environmental Advocacy Committee at her children's school.

Originally from the small rural town of Preston, Connecticut, Elizabeth received a B.S. from Eastern Connecticut State University as well as a certificate in Nutrition Fundamentals from Cornell University to augment her ever-expanding knowledge of diet and nutrition. She lives in Santa Cruz, California, with her husband and two children.

Beanalicious Living is her first book. Readers can connect with Elizabeth via her website **www.ElizabethBorelli.com**.

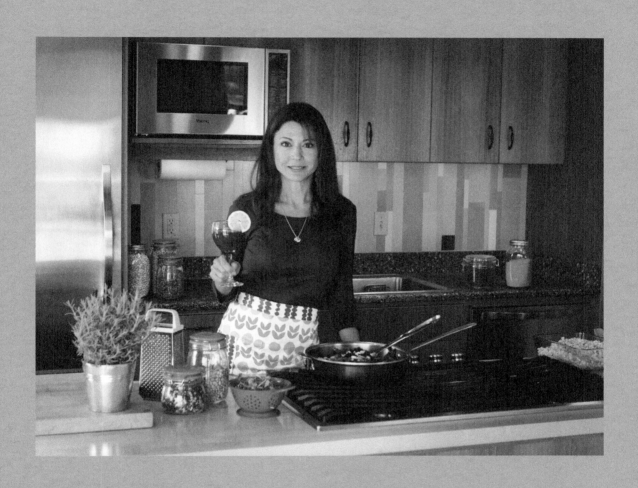

CPSIA information can be obtained at www.ICGtesting.com
Printed in the USA
BVOW11s0807291113

337662BV00001B/1/P

9 781939 288196